Mohamed Abdel-Raheem
Taghreed Khudhur Muhammed

Microorganisms and Insects Used in Forensic Detection

Mohamed Abdel-Raheem
Taghreed Khudhur Muhammed

Microorganisms and Insects Used in Forensic Detection

Noor Publishing

Cover image: www.ingimage.com

Publisher:
Noor Publishing
is a trademark of
Dodo Books Indian Ocean Ltd. and OmniScriptum S.R.L publishing group

120 High Road, East Finchley, London, N2 9ED, United Kingdom
Str. Armeneasca 28/1, office 1, Chisinau MD-2012, Republic of Moldova, Europe
Managing Directors: Ieva Konstantinova, Victoria Ursu
info@omniscriptum.com

Printed at: see last page
ISBN: 978-620-8-87035-5

Microorganisms and Insects Used in Forensic Detection

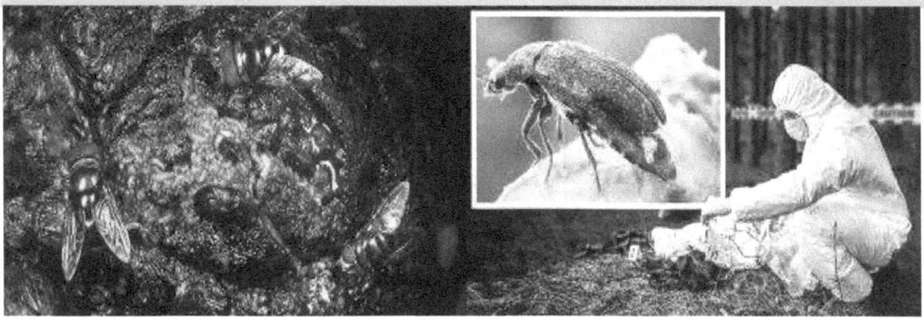

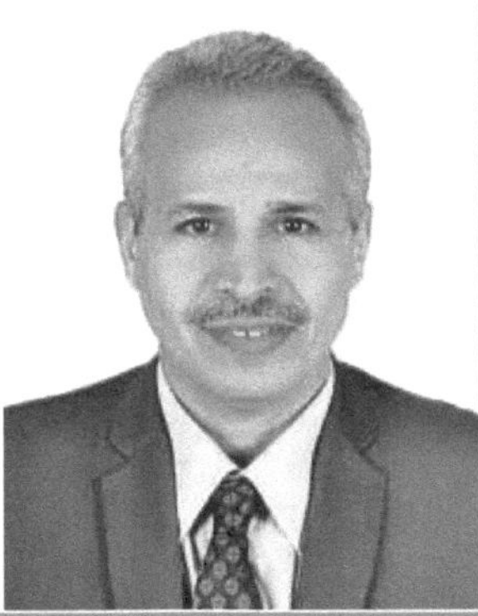

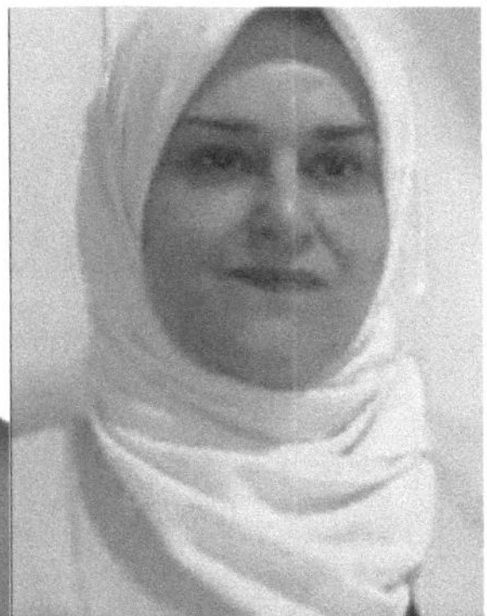

By

Prof. Dr. Mohamed Abdel-Raheem

Prof. Dr. Taghreed Khudhur Muhammed

(2025)

Microorganisms and Insects Used in Forensic Detection

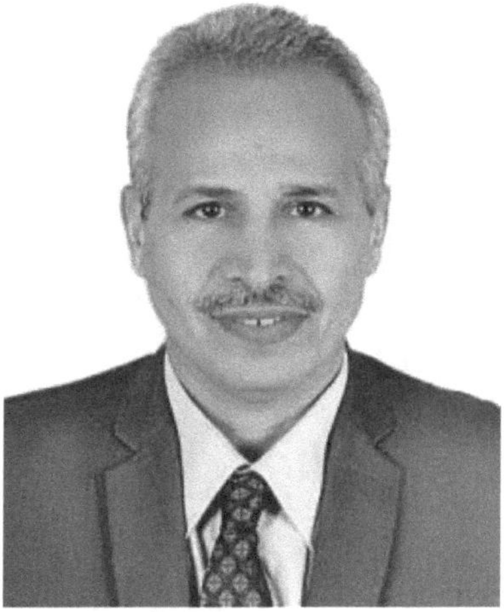

Prof. Dr. Mohamed Abdel-Raheem Ali Abdel-Raheem

Professor of Biological Control

Pests & Plant Protection Department

Agricultural and Biological Research Institute

National Research Centre.

Microorganisms and Insects Used in Forensic Detection

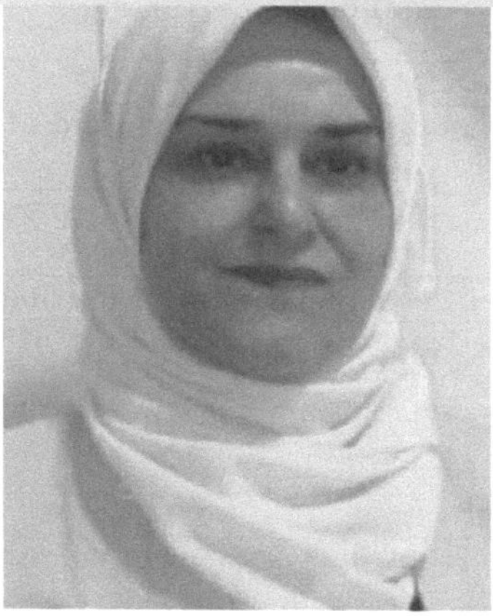

Prof. Dr. Taghreed Khudhur Muhammed

Microbiology, Bacterial Toxicology, Technical

Medical Institute, Al-Mansour - Middle Technical

Content list

Subject	Page
Introduction	6
Incorporation of the microbiome into the field of forensic sciences	17
Analysis of the microbiome and personalized identification.	20
Interest in the Study of Biological Fluids Microbiomes	24
Utilizing Microbiome Analysis for Estimation of the Post-Mortem Interval (PMI)	34
Microbiomes	38
Factors that impact the analysis of microbiome	40
Potential Bacterial biomarkers for insect colonization in Forensic Cases	48
Bacterial specific *gyr*B primers	52
Wohlfahrtiimonas chitiniclastica in insect immature stages	54
Ignatzschineria indica in insect immature stages	57
Isolation and identification of virulent bacteria from forensic flies	67
Studying the colonization patterns of insects and microbial communities in buried remains of forensic significance	90
Quantitative polymerase chain reaction (qPCR)	98
Diptera and Coleoptera succession	105
16S rRNA Illumina MiSeq characterization of insect and rat small intestine tissues	107
Insect dynamics on buried rat carcasses	120
Insect microbiome	123
In search of bacterial PMI biomarkers	126
Forensic Entomology	129
Types of forensic entomology	141
Insects as a forensic indicator in crime investigation	144
Dipteran insect shows complete metamorphosis	146
Insects' collection, entomological preservation methods, simulation and rearing	150

Wildlife Forensic Entomology	**154**
Concepts, Procedures and Techniques Used by Forensic Entomologists and Proxies	**158**
Forensic Entomology for Crime Scene Investigations	**160**
Forensic Entomology in Crime	**165**
Crime Scene and Health Pathology Facility	**175**
Preservation of Insects	**184**
Preparation of Insects at the Crime Scene for Rearing Purposes	**187**
Examining Larvae and Full Puparia for Age Determination	**191**
Insect Successional Studies	**203**
Identification of Diptera Puparia in Forensic and Archeo-Funerary Contexts	**204**
Definition, Structure, and Formation of Puparia	**209**
DNA-Based Approach	**215**
Fragmentation and Chemical Modifications	**218**
Methodology Remarks	**222**
Application in forensics	**230**
Future perspectives	**239**
Artificial Intelligence in the Field of Forensic Biology	**240**
Conclusions	**243**
References	**247**

Introduction

The primary aim of forensic sciences is to identify evidence in a crime scene with the purpose of reconstructing the events that transpired. Traditional examples of such evidence include DNA and fingerprints, although they are not without their limitations and may not always provide conclusive information. A relatively new type of evidence that has gained importance is the microbiome. With the backing of the Human Microbiome Project, the characteristics of microbial communities show considerable promise in the field of forensics. These communities are exceptionally precise and can be utilized to distinguish and categorize the specific body site from which a human biological sample originated. The microbiota present on the skin is particularly distinct and varies among individuals, making it a potential tool for identification purposes. Furthermore, the potential for microbial communities to be transferred onto common objects has also been investigated. Additional applications of microbiome analysis in forensics include determining the time of death and studying soil communities. However, a key challenge lies in the fact that the microbiome is subject to change over time and can be influenced by various environmental and lifestyle factors.

In many cases of violent criminal behaviour, the perpetrator frequently seeks to conceal the crime and dispose of the victim's body by burying it, typically in shallow graves, due to the weight and size of human bodies. Once buried, the remains are exposed to a range of elements that can affect the process of decomposition and consequently the estimation of the postmortem interval (PMI). These elements may encompass abiotic elements such as soil pH, temperature, composition, and moisture levels, as well as biotic factors like the presence of environmental microbial communities and availability to insect colonizers [1,2].

Given the impact of living organisms on the decomposition process, it is essential to consider the roles of microbes and insects when determining the post-mortem interval (PMI) for buried bodies. Existing research on insect and bacterial species involved in decomposition has mostly focused on surface remains, prompting this study to explore the decomposition of buried rat carcasses as a model for human cadavers [3-11].

Numerous studies have been conducted in various countries such as Great Britain, Poland, Australia, Argentina, the United States of America, Canada, Germany, and South Africa to investigate the decomposition process of buried remains. The majority of these studies utilized human cadavers and pig carcasses, with a small number incorporating juvenile rat and sheep carcasses as experimental models, although comprehensive analyses of both bacterial and insect communities were lacking. These investigations examined a range of decomposition-related topics, including initial observations of decay processes in different soil types, patterns of necrophagous insect species colonization, and recent efforts to characterize the structure of the decomposition necrobiome for forensic purposes [12-32].

The process of carcass decomposition in the soil is distinct from surface remains, which typically undergo a series of identifiable stages including fresh, bloat, active decay, advanced decay, and ultimately skeletal remains. Buried remains, like surface remains, can also progress through defined stages of decomposition. This begins with the fresh stage, characterized by visible swelling of the abdomen. Subsequently, the remains enter primary and secondary bloat stages, marked by gas accumulation and pungent odours. Eventually, as the abdomen deflates, the remains move into the active decay stage where decomposer and scavenger communities are still active in breaking down tissues. With continued degradation, the remains transition into the advanced decay stage where the abdomen and rib cage collapse, flesh liquefies or disappears, and adipocere formation may be evident as the remains progress towards the skeletal stage [33,34].

Additionally, the decomposition of surface and buried remains is significantly influenced by taphonomic elements including ante mortem conditions (such as covering, clothing, and wounds), environmental factors like the characteristics of the grave and soil, seasonal variations, temperature, and the presence of insects and scavengers [33-35].

Temperature fluctuation is a key factor in the decomposition of carcasses, with a temperature range of 20 to 40 degrees Celsius being ideal for tissue breakdown, especially at 37 degrees Celsius. Extreme temperatures outside of this range, below 10 degrees Celsius or above 40 degrees Celsius, can hinder the decomposition process. Furthermore, variations in climate patterns can impact insect activity and the potential for carcass colonization in soil. Decomposition in buried settings is also influenced by the presence of oxygen, with limited quantities potentially altering the composition and structure of microbial communities involved in decomposition, as well as delaying the process by affecting insect colonization [29,30].

When examining a buried location, it is essential to take into account the various environmental factors such as depth, geographic location, season, and weather conditions. Additionally, the composition and chemical makeup of the soil plays a crucial role in the decomposition process and must not be overlooked [13].

Moreover, the composition of the soil-dwelling necrophagous entomofauna differs significantly from that found on the surface, with variations in the abundance and diversity of dominant families. Notably, specimens from the Phoridae and Muscidae families are often discovered in buried carcasses, in contrast to the Calliphoridae family members that typically colonize surface remains as primary and predominant colonizers. The process of colonization begins when necrophagous insects deposit eggs on the soil surface or navigate through the soil to access the carcass, a behaviour that can be influenced by factors such as season, temperature, soil texture, and burial depth. Previous studies have consistently identified Phoridae, Muscidae, and Sarcophagidae as the primary species recovered from buried remains. However, there is a limited number of case reports documenting the necrophagous entomofauna associated with buried bodies, as most research tends to focus on exhumation studies [30-39].

Additionally, the developing realm of forensic microbiology has strived to address specific challenges faced in determining the postmortem interval by leveraging predictable alterations in the microbial composition. These research efforts centre on analyzing the necrobiome structure of vertebrate remains, monitoring changes in microbial communities as decomposition occurs, and examining the microbial and fungal populations in the surrounding soil linked to the decaying carcass [40-47].

Overall, forensic microbiology aims to enhance the field of forensic entomology by presenting an additional method for estimating postmortem intervals through similar principles. However, research on the microbiome of decomposition and insect microbiome primarily concentrates on surface remains, with less emphasis on buried remains. These initial investigations were essential in understanding the decomposition process, but they were conducted either in controlled laboratory settings or solely explored the variety of soil-related bacterial communities [47- 50].

The current knowledge indicates that soil, host-associated, and insect-associated microbial communities undergo changes as decomposition progresses. The focus of forensic research is on the ability to monitor these changes over time, with many studies aiming to identify overall community changes and specific variations in certain members that could serve as indicators of postmortem interval. A recent study examining specific taxa within the human gut microbiome revealed that certain taxa can be traced throughout the decomposition process. For instance, *Bacteroides* sp., *Lactobacillus* sp., and *Bifidobacterium* sp. were monitored using qPCR as potential quantitative markers of postmortem interval during human cadaver decomposition. Other studies on phylum Firmicutes have concentrated on quantitative analysis of water samples or the broader intestinal microbiota [51-53].

In order to gain a deeper understanding of the contributions of insects and microbes in the decomposition of buried remains and their relevance to estimating the postmortem interval, this study offers a comprehensive examination of both insects and bacteria as primary decomposers and the potential environmental factors impacting the process. The utilization of rat carcasses as substitutes for human remains allowed for the observation of changes in insect behaviour and microbial communities. Rat carcasses serve as widely accepted animal models in clinical human research, providing a level of reproducibility and ease of sampling not readily achievable with human specimens. Furthermore, previous forensic studies have successfully utilized rodents due to the similarities in decomposition processes and microbial makeup between rat carcasses and human cadavers [53-59].

The research was conducted in two 30-day time periods in the spring and summer months (March and June) within a temperate continental climate region in Eastern Europe (specifically Bucharest, Romania). The primary goals of this investigation were to qualitatively and quantitatively evaluate the necrophagous insect fauna and microbiome present during the decomposition of buried rat carcasses, as well as to explore the impact of environmental variables on the decomposition process while also analyzing the colonization patterns of key decomposers. Understanding the behaviour of necrophagous insect species in relation to colonization and the bacterial communities associated with carcasses and insects is crucial for accurately estimating the postmortem interval for buried remains [60].

Trace evidence is typically described as remaining evidence from a previous event or action by an event or an agent. Examination of the different materials found at a crime scene is a crucial aspect of investigations, as it has the potential to uncover the presence or connections between individuals, or between individuals and an object or location. These indicators of criminal activity are generally divided into three main categories: digital forensics, physics and chemistry, and human identification. Alphonse Bertillon, a renowned French forensic scientist, was the first to utilize microorganisms as trace evidence and determine their source. He studied approximately 500,000 microbes/m^3 and 88,000 microbes in various locations in Paris (Figure 1) [61, 62].

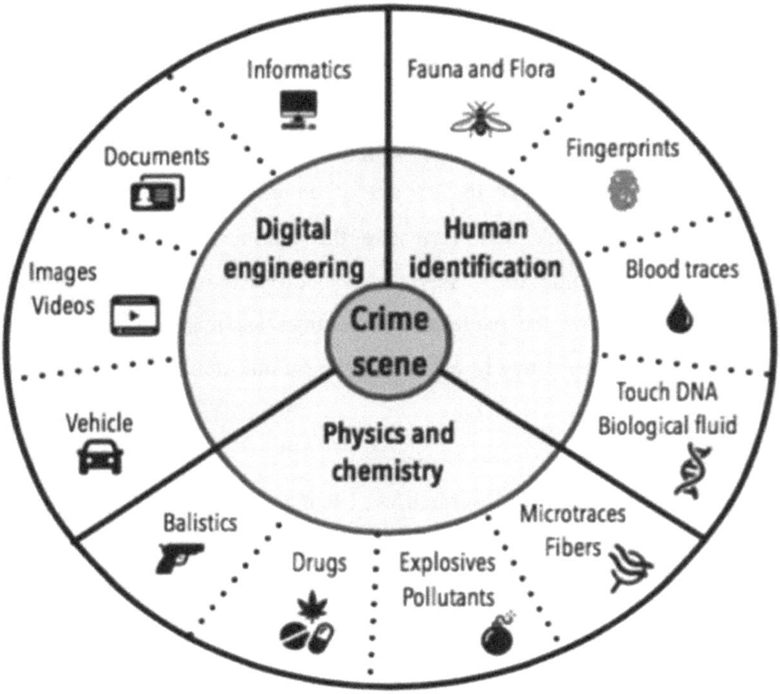

Figure 1: There are certain pieces of evidence that may be discovered at the scene of a crime [61]

In criminal investigations, any item that can be linked to the scene of the crime may serve as evidence. Physical evidence plays a critical role in providing essential information for victim, suspect, or witness statements. The collection of DNA and fingerprints offers the benefit of being possible on various surfaces. In the field of forensic science, the processes of creating, obtaining samples, and analyzing trace evidence have been conceptualized by Inman and Rudin, who have identified six key principles: divisibility, transfer, classification, identification, association, and reconstruction [63, 64].

Crime scene analysis comprises three distinct levels: the source, the activity, and the offense. At the source level, experts focus on determining the material origin of trace evidence in order to establish an individual profile and identify potential suspects present at the scene. The activity level involves developing theories on the mechanisms and actions that resulted in the deposition of the trace evidence, facilitating the reconstruction of the sequence of events that transpired. The final level, the offense, falls within the jurisdiction of magistrates and involves a comprehensive assessment of the criminal actions, including the significance of the evidence and contextual elements or motives, to ascertain culpability and the reasons behind the crime (Figure 2).

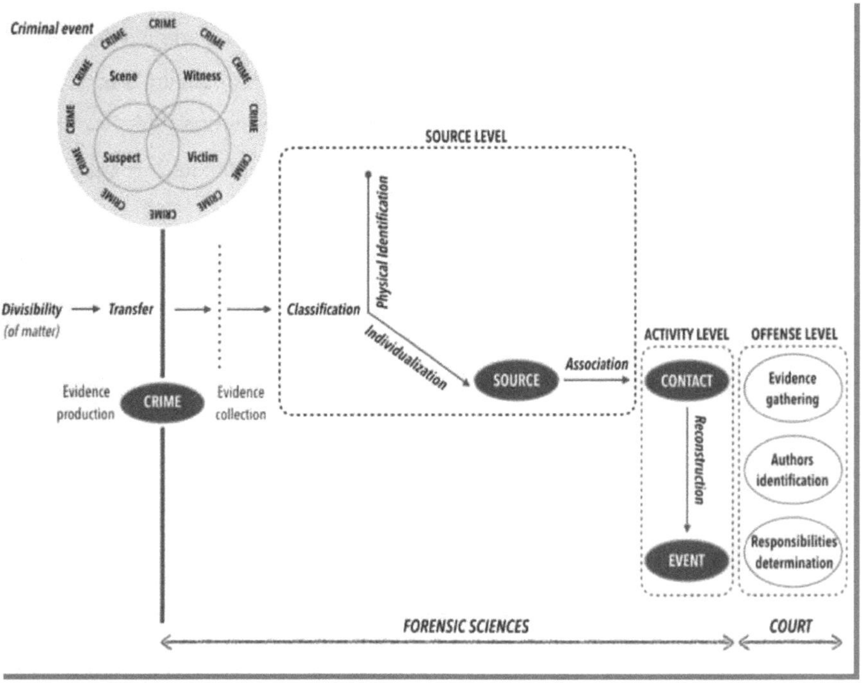

Figure 2: The foundational tenets of forensic science [64]

Historically, the identification of suspects has relied upon a combination of DNA analysis and fingerprinting. However, these methods are not without their drawbacks: DNA samples may be degraded, contaminated, or insufficient in quantity for accurate interpretation, while fingerprints can be incomplete or overlapping. Furthermore, trace amounts of bodily fluids are often present in limited quantities and may be mixed, presenting challenges in their definitive identification [65, 66].

In order to ascertain the sequence of events at the crime scene, it is crucial to establish the existence and source of biological evidence. The existing genetic analysis, which relies on Short Tandem Repeat (STR) sequences, can provide an individual's genetic profile but falls short in determining the manner in which the trace was left behind. Identifying the source of biological fluids is instrumental in addressing this issue. Various presumptive or confirmatory tests, whether chemical or immunological, are currently employed to detect biological fluids such as saliva, blood, or sperm. Nevertheless, these tests have constraints in terms of sensitivity and/or specificity [66-68].

Alternative methods used for the prediction and differentiation of body fluids include mRNA, miRNA, and epigenetic markers such as methylation levels of GpC islands. Various markers, such as ankyrin 1 for blood, protamines for semen, and histatin for saliva, have been identified for common forensic biological fluids. These markers can be easily recovered from different surfaces and exhibit relative stability in body fluids. The main approach involves determining the number of transcripts for each body fluid by analyzing the total DNA or RNA, yet these methods may lack specificity. Additionally, mRNA markers can be influenced by various factors including age, diet, and health status. MiRNA have emerged as a promising alternative due to their high stability, even in post-mortem samples, and some are specific to humans. However, a drawback of miRNA markers is their lack of specificity to a particular body fluid or part. Despite this limitation, several studies have identified specific markers for peripheral blood, semen, and vaginal epithelium [67-70].

Epigenetic investigations primarily rely on the analysis of DNA methylation. Discrepancies in epigenetic patterns within GpC islands have been noted across various biological fluids, and can be identified through PCR and/or bisulfite conversion. The concurrent utilization of both techniques appears to offer the most effective approach [69].

The advancement of next-generation sequencing (NGS) technologies, which incorporate miniaturization and enhanced performance has significantly decreased the time required for sequencing one or more genomes. These technologies not only enable the identification of single or multiple traces but also provide valuable additional information for forensic investigations. Despite these improvements in DNA analysis, there remains a number of unsolved criminal cases, underscoring the importance of enhancing the evidential elements to link perpetrators to crime scenes. These NGS technologies have the potential to be utilized in studying the human microbiota in various organs. Consequently, the emergence of microbiota analysis offers an encouraging alternative to current forensic analysis methods due to the ubiquitous presence of bacteria throughout the body, each individual possessing a unique microbiota [71].

Incorporation of the microbiome into the field of forensic sciences

Microbiome analysis used in forensics offers significant advantages due to the diversity and wide prevalence of microbial communities unique to each individual. The human microbiota comprises 10-100 trillion symbiotic microbial cells specific to each person, with various bacterial communities present at different body sites as revealed by research. For instance, the mouth contains approximately 200 species, while the intestinal tract harbors about 400 species. Furthermore, the circular form and membrane of bacterial DNA provide it with greater resistance to degradation compared to human DNA. This feature enables techniques commonly employed in medical analysis to be utilized in forensic investigations, resulting in enhanced information beyond DNA analysis alone. While microbiome analysis is increasingly utilized in medical, public health, ecological, and industrial settings, its application in forensics is a nascent tool with limited integration in criminal investigations [72-79].

The human skin harbours a diverse cutaneous microbiota, which can readily be transferred to various surfaces or objects. These microbial communities are capable of persisting on touched surfaces for extended periods due to bacteria's resilience to environmental stressors such as humidity, temperature, and ultraviolet radiation. An individual's lifestyle choices, such as diet, living conditions, health status, smoking habits, and pet ownership, can influence the composition of their microbiome. As a result, there is continuous interaction between humans and their surroundings, leading to microbial exchanges. Specific bacteria can be retrieved from classrooms, living spaces, and work environments to ascertain an individual's presence. Analyzing an individual's personal microbiome can potentially link them to a crime scene or the victim through the identification of their bacterial community [80-82].

The foundation of microbial forensics lies in the characterization of microorganisms in a given sample, achieved through establishing the correlation between the presence of bacterial communities and the specific anatomical site or tissue under scrutiny. The inaugural instance of its application occurred following a bioterrorist incident involving *Bacillus anthracis* in the United States, just one week after the 11 September attacks. The spores of this particular species were enclosed in envelopes and dispatched to the premises of American senators and media outlets. An investigation was launched by the Federal Bureau of Investigation (FBI) employing microbial forensics to pinpoint the individual responsible. The inquiry proceeded over an extended period due to the inadequacy of available analysis methodologies, including the lack of reference strains and the challenge of evaluating the probative value of the evidence. The FBI formally concluded its investigation in the year 2011 [76,83]. Microbial forensics was primarily utilized in this instance to identify pathogens utilized as biological weapons or to track the spread of certain human viruses among perpetrators. Initial microbial analyses in the field of forensics have verified the existence or non-existence of bacterial strains to establish distinct indicators. Six particular microbial indicators were emphasized for the differentiation of vaginal, oral, and faecal specimens. Nevertheless, these investigations employed a limited number of markers and samples, thus lacking representation of actuality, leading to numerous instances of inaccurate positive and negative results [84].

Many current research studies have since examined the potential applications of microbiome analysis. This publication provides a comprehensive examination of the primary methodologies and findings generated from the study of microbial communities (Figure 3) [84].

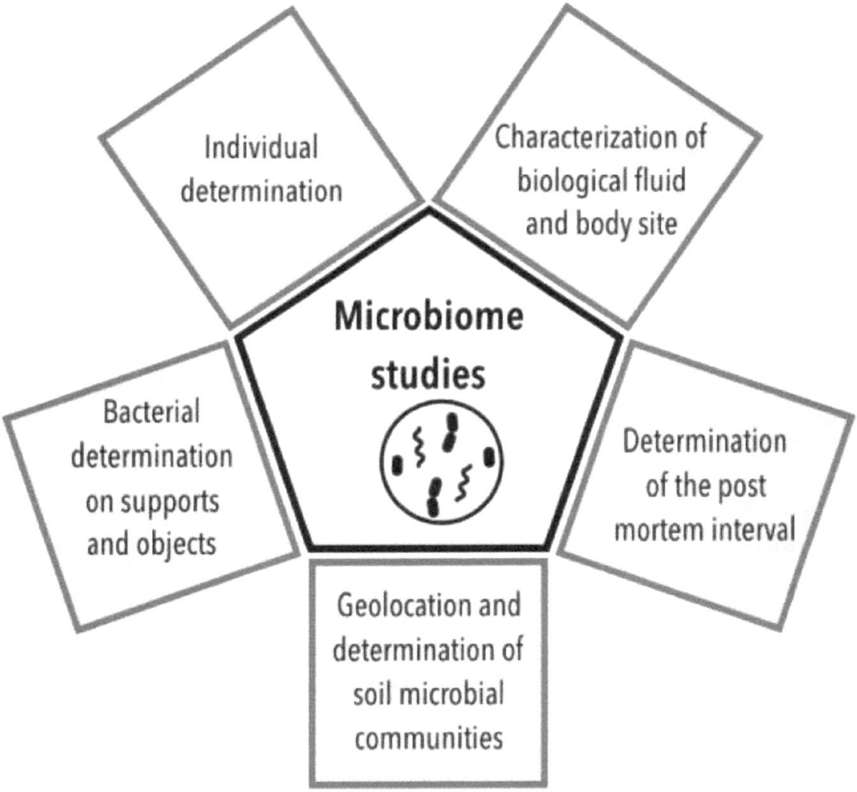

Figure 3: Microbiome analysis toolbox [84].

Analysis of the microbiome and personalized identification

The microbial composition in various areas of the body appears to be distinct and consistent over time. The skin serves as a primary defense barrier against pathogens. Despite this, the skin is not completely free of microorganisms, with approximately 10^7 cells/cm^2 consisting mainly of bacteria, along with viruses, fungi, and dust mites. Consequently, the bacterial populations on the skin are diverse, dynamic, and differ across different regions of the skin's surface. For instance, only 13% of bacteria in the palm are shared among individuals [85].

The maintenance of skin equilibrium is largely attributed to these bacterial communities, though the presence of other less common species also contributes to the unique nature of the skin microbiota. Notably, the composition of skin communities varies significantly more than those in the gut or oral cavity due to greater exposure to environmental fluctuations [85-88].

Delineation of the Fundamental Microbial Community

While each person possesses a distinct bacterial composition, there are commonalities among individuals delineated by the core microbiome. This core microbiome represents bacterial communities shared by all individuals and plays a crucial role in various functions within the human body. Schmedes *et al.* conducted research on the connection between different skin sites and their respective hosts by pinpointing specific bacterial markers. They identified ten key bacterial species that are significant for forensic analyses, with *Cutibacterium* (formerly *Propionibacterium*) acnes being prevalent in all samples. The presence or absence of this bacterium could be a determining factor in identifying whether a sample is of skin origin. It is important to note, however, that the aforementioned study was not carried out in a forensic setting [89, 90].

The researchers concluded their investigation by utilizing hidskinPlex markers, which include both common and unique markers, to discern skin microbiomes among various individuals. This innovative sequencing technique shows potential in its capability to differentiate between distinct body regions. In their research, Costello *et al.* analyzed the diversity of microbial populations across various body regions by collecting samples from diverse locations on the skin. Each specific body region exhibited a consistent and unique core microbiome within individuals over time. Nevertheless, the differences between individuals were more pronounced than the variations within the same individual, and the identification of the core microbiome relied on the specific body region being examined [91].

Example of Specific Bacterial Communities

Hands are a crucial element in forensic analysis. Research has examined the typical microbial makeup of hands and how it can change and transfer onto surfaces. Hands harbour a distinctive microbiome consisting of 8-24 primary bacteria families and approximately 150 species. The dominant species found on hands are *Micrococcus* and *Staphylococcus* [92, 93].

However, while fingerprints remain consistent over time, the microbiota found on hands experience fluctuations and are consequently less stable. Various internal and external physiological factors of the hands play a role in determining the stability of this microbial community. Age and gender both play a significant role in influencing the composition of microorganisms. Children's hands tend to have a higher presence of Firmicutes species, whereas adults' hands are more likely to harbour Propionibacteria. Additionally, there is a greater bacterial diversity present on women's hands compared to men's. This disparity may be attributed to differences in skin pH between males and females or hormonal variations in the hands. Further research is essential to determine the longevity of microbial populations on hands [94, 95].

Personal Microbial Cloud

Meadow *et al.* conducted a study on the concept of the "personal microbial cloud," which refers to the unique microbial communities that surround an individual, similar to a personal aerosol. This study aimed to identify a human microbiome signal by analyzing the microbial communities present in the air around individuals. The researchers placed participants in a sterile room with controlled conditions, such as pressure, temperature, and air filtration, and collected air filters to determine individual-specific microbial communities. The results showed that each participant emitted a distinct microbial signal, which was directly linked to airborne particles in the surrounding air. Despite certain limitations in the methodology, such as the number of participants, the amount of analyzed particles, ambient conditions, time spent in the room, and the microbial background, this approach provides valuable insights into evaluating skin microbiota in a controlled environment [96].

Cross Transfer between Individuals

Research has examined the relationship between the human microbiome and personal belongings. When conducting forensic analysis, it is essential to determine whether the transfer of microbes was from direct contact between a person and an object, or indirect contact between a person, an object, and another person. The microbial communities found on humans can consist of a variety of microorganisms. It is crucial to ascertain whether these microorganisms originate from a singular source or if there has been a transfer from an object, another individual, or a different area of the body. Neckovic *et al.* conducted a study on both direct transfer of microbes through a handshake and indirect transfer through an intermediary substrate, such as a previously touched object or surface [97].

During a period of three days, various materials such as paper, cotton fabric, and glass were tested after being touched by different individuals living separately. A control sample was also taken from the right finger of each person. Their findings revealed that both types of transfers affected the microbial communities present. The challenge lay in quantifying this transfer and assessing its longevity. This raised doubts about the ability to link a person to an object, though it could prove valuable in instances of sexual assault involving significant skin contact. To implement this approach in forensic science, precautions must be taken to prevent contamination hazards [97].

Interest in the Study of Biological Fluids Microbiomes

The genetic analysis of Short Tandem Repeat (STR) polymorphisms provides information about an individual's genetic makeup but does not reveal the manner in which traces are left at a specific location. Identifying body fluids is crucial in forensic inquiries as it aids in reconstructing events that transpired at a crime scene. For instance, in instances of bite marks, detecting the suspect's saliva is pertinent, and in cases of alleged sexual assault, determining vaginal microbial communities is essential. The placement of biological samples can provide insight into the presence or absence of consent in sexual interactions and corroborate the accounts of victims or suspects [97].

Saliva

Saliva is a ubiquitous biological fluid that can be found on various surfaces at a crime scene as a result of actions such as kissing, biting, or licking. It is known to contain an average of 500 million bacterial cells/mL and approximately 700 different bacterial species. The oral cavity serves as the primary gateway for microorganisms to enter the digestive system, with the teeth, tongue, and cheek providing conducive environments for microbial colonization. The oral environment experiences a notable degree of variability due to regular exposure to external factors [98].

Various external influences such as tobacco, drugs, and cosmetic products can impact the composition of the oral microbiota. Limited research has been conducted on the long-term stability and dynamics of the oral microbiome. Nevertheless, a core microbiota in saliva has been identified, hinting at some degree of individualized stability. While this stability may be evident in the short term, it is subject to variation over extended periods [98].

Jung *et al.* have introduced a novel tool for saliva identification utilizing multiplex real-time PCR, with a focus on three oral bacterial markers. The method demonstrated high specificity, as only a single saliva marker was detected in each fecal sample, and exhibited sensitivity in detecting markers even with small amounts of saliva up to 14 weeks post-collection. These distinct oral bacteria were present in 91.4% of the samples, with DNA concentrations detected at minute levels (0.13 ng of total DNA). The researchers noted that tooth brushing had minimal impact on the presence of these specific markers. Although microbial community detection was slightly compromised on items such as cigarettes, mugs, forks, and bite marks following brushing, all samples still yielded positive results. Additionally, prolonged storage did not hinder the detection of markers. Remarkably, no cell lysis treatment was deemed necessary, permitting further analysis of the sample to ascertain a genetic profile of the individual under scrutiny [99].

Leake *et al.* conducted an analysis of the variations of saliva at both the inter- and intra-individual levels. They collected saliva samples from two healthy adults at various intervals and utilized three specific targets (*rpo*B gene 1 for *Streptococcus*, *rpo*B gene 2 for other bacteria, and 16S rRNA) to enhance identification accuracy. Their study illustrated the distinct specificity of salivary microbiota, enabling the differentiation between the two individuals. However, the limited number of volunteers in this research indicates the necessity for a larger-scale study to validate the utility of this method [77]

Vaginal Secretions

Identification of vaginal fluids plays a crucial role in cases of sexual assault. The primary dominant communities found in healthy human vaginal secretions are *Lactobacillus* species, which serve to defend women against harmful pathogens and opportunistic infections. The microbial composition of vaginal samples remains relatively consistent regardless of the stage of the female menstrual cycle or pregnancy. Conditions like vaginosis may disrupt the equilibrium of the "normal" vaginal microbiota, leading to dysbiosis [100-102].

Giampaoli *et al.* conducted an analysis on swabs taken from vaginal, oral, and faecal areas, as well as forensic samples from female genital regions, utilizing real-time PCR. The results aligned with the specific body site from which the samples were collected, although there were instances where vaginal bacteria were also detected in faecal samples. Their examination extended to mixtures of different samples, revealing no significant alteration to the typical vaginal flora or complicating the interpretation of these intricate samples. These findings hold promise in the realm of distinguishing individuals through microbiota-based approaches in instances of sexual assault or violence. Furthermore, the researchers utilized a consistent extraction protocol for both microbial communities and STR analysis, eliminating the necessity for multiple samples in forensic investigations.

Doi *et al.* devised a technique for detecting *Lactobacillus* in vaginal secretions through real-time PCR. They formulated a *Lactobacillus* primer based on the alignment of sequences from 16S RNA across various *Lactobacillus* species. This methodology effectively differentiated vaginal secretions, characterized by low cycle threshold (Ct) values, from other bodily fluids [103].

Blood Samples

Diez Lopez and colleagues conducted a study to classify blood, a common fluid encountered in crime scenes, by utilizing 16S rRNA gene sequencing. They were able to identify four distinct types of blood: menstrual blood, venous blood, nasal blood, and blood originating from skin epithelium. Menstrual blood samples stood out due to the prevalence of *Lactobacillus* species, yet results could be influenced by the phase of the menstrual cycle and potential vaginal infections. Venous blood exhibited generic components related to human host proteins, with minimal bacterial presence reflecting the typically sterile nature of blood in a healthy individual. Nasal blood classification was less definitive, attributed to the potential dilution of microorganisms from nasal blowing, but hints of nasal microbiota bacteria suggested the blood's source. Meanwhile, the detection of microorganisms from cutaneous microbiota aided in distinguishing blood from skin epithelium. The efficacy of this taxonomic screening approach should be assessed in larger-scale studies [104].

Fecal Material

Fecal samples serve as a reliable representation of the gut microbiota, with significantly higher levels of bacteria compared to other types of samples. However, exposing these predominantly anaerobic microorganisms to aerobic conditions can complicate the process of microbiota determination. The gut microbiota is conventionally dominated by two main phyla, Firmicutes and Bacteroidetes, which form the core microbiome of the intestines. While these bacterial communities tend to be stable, substantial variability at the species level has been documented among individuals, facilitating the differentiation of even monozygotic twins through microbiome analysis. The full diversity of the gut microbiota typically becomes established by around the age of 4, with its composition subject to influences such as genetics, health status, age, lifestyle choices, dietary habits, environmental factors, and exposure to various treatments. Notably, the administration of antibiotics has been shown to significantly impact gut microbial communities. In essence, the gut microbiota is often likened to a unique digital fingerprint [105-107].

Scalp and Pubic Hairs

Hair is often found at crime scenes, but the amount of nuclear DNA is usually insufficient for reliable genetic profiling. The microbial communities found on hair shafts are unique and specific to each individual. Tridico *et al.* conducted a study using metagenomic approaches to analyze hair, focusing on distinguishing between scalp and pubic hairs based on microbial composition, identifying individuals based on colonizing microorganisms, and studying the persistence of hair bacterial communities over time. The microbial composition of pubic hair was found to be relatively stable and less affected by environmental factors compared to scalp hair, although sexual activity can alter these microbial populations. Female pubic hair often harbours *Lactobacillus* sp., which acts as a protective barrier against other microorganisms and distinguishes between male and female pubic hair. No significant differences were observed in microbial communities between male and female scalp hair, but scalp hair microbiota appeared to be more sensitive to environmental changes compared to pubic hair [108].

Brinkac *et al.* interestingly observed that the geographical origin, specifically different states in the USA, had an impact on the composition of hair microbiota, thus indicating that hair samples could be utilized effectively in forensic analysis.

The authors also pointed out that certain characteristics of hair, such as its length, were influential in determining the diversity of microbes present [109].

In a study by Williams *et al.*, samples from the pubic hairs of sexually active couples were examined. It was found that male samples predominantly contained *Corynebacterium* species, while female samples contained *Lactobacillus* species, indicating a distinct microbial composition based on gender. The study also noted a varied mix of microbial communities in cases of sexual activity, with an increase in similarity between individual microbial communities corresponding to the frequency of sexual encounters. Additionally, it was discovered that couples shared a similar hair microbiome (pubic and ears), although this was not directly correlated with sexual activity[108].

Furthermore, the potential transfer of microbes and any links between a victim and an assailant were explored. By creating a hypothetical scenario involving a victim, her partner, and an unknown assailant, Williams *et al.* were able to generate a new microbial profile attributed to the assailant. However, the formal identification of this individual based on microbial evidence alone was deemed unattainable. Nevertheless, this technique may prove to be useful in narrowing down potential suspects in criminal investigations [109].

Sperm Sample

The microbiome present in testicular sperm is characterized by a low biomass yet significant contamination, while the microbiome in semen is characterized by a diverse and abundant composition. Baud *et al.* conducted a study on the composition of seminal fluid and its impact on sperm characteristics, revealing that the recovered microbial communities were specific to sperm. Certain bacterial genera such as *Lactobacillus* and *Staphylococcus* were found to be associated with normal sperm, akin to vaginal and cutaneous microbiota. The composition of this microbiota did not show a direct correlation with sperm quality. However, the presence of pathogenic bacteria such as *Ureaplasma urealyticum*, *Mycoplasma hominis*, and *Prevotella* sp. had a detrimental effect on semen quality. This finding could hold promise for forensic investigations where the absence of spermatozoa poses a challenge [110-112].

Other Samples

Quaak *et al.* conducted a study examining various biological samples such as saliva, feces, penile swabs, and hand swabs in order to distinguish between the microbial populations present in each. They found that oral and fecal samples exhibited a greater diversity of microorganisms compared to vaginal and skin samples. Unique species such as *Lactobacillus* and *Streptococcus salivarius* were identified in vaginal and oral microbial communities, respectively. It is worth noting that these species were also detected in other sample types. Remarkably, the abundance of each species was distinctive enough to pinpoint the origin of the sample. Understanding the fundamental microbiome composition in different bodily fluids or regions appears to be a crucial initial finding in forensic inquiries [113]

Determining the microbiome present on various surfaces and items

Microbial research can utilize trace DNA found on items such as eyeglasses, cell phones, and doorknobs. The correlation between the bacteria present in the human skin microbiome and that found on various surfaces or objects underscores the influence of the human microbiome on the microbial composition in different settings, such as residences, workplaces, and urban areas. While there have been extensive studies on the fluctuating nature of the microbiome, less focus has been placed on the stability of external samples taken from humans. These investigations could be crucial in forensic science for determining the origin of bodily fluids discovered at crime scenes, as these samples may have been impacted by exposure to natural human environments, storage conditions, and laboratory procedures [82].

Mobile Phones

Cellular devices are frequently utilized on a daily basis and have the capability to provide data concerning location or indicators of health. Numerous research studies have indicated that microbial populations originating from the skin can be detected on mobile phones. Specimens collected from the thumb, fingers of the dominant hand, and the touchscreen of smartphones revealed that bacterial populations were associated with human body regions. Interestingly, a notable discrepancy was observed between males and females; the composition of bacterial communities on the fingers of women closely resembled that of their phones, whereas in men, it differed. Lax *et al.* established that microorganisms recovered from the rear of phones were consistent with microbial communities found on hands, while microorganisms present on the front of phones corresponded to the facial microbiota. Additionally, the microbial compositions on phones demonstrated instability, largely attributed to the rapid turnover of microorganisms on the individual's hands. It is important to underscore that the samples were collected within a timeframe of less than 3 days post-deposit, rendering this investigation challenging to apply within forensic science contexts [114, 115].

Keyboards and Mice

Fierer and colleagues conducted an assessment of the microbial communities found on computer keyboards and mice in relation to those of the users. The similarity in bacterial populations on both the devices and the users' fingers indicates the presence of a distinct bacterial profile unique to each individual. The impact of storage conditions on the microbial communities of these objects was found to have minimal effect on the composition of bacterial populations. [80].

Shoes

In order to assess the impact of geographical location on microbial populations, Lax *et al.* collected samples from the shoes of three individuals residing in distinct municipalities within the United States and Canada, in conjunction with soil samples. The researchers noted a substantial divergence among the microbial communities present on the participants' shoes, presumably attributable to the unique microbiome of each shoe. Not surprisingly, the majority of microorganisms found on the shoes originated from the soil. Conversely, the microbial communities on shoes could potentially be transferred onto soil, thereby impacting the microbial populations on the floor. This transfer of microorganisms appeared to occur regardless of the material composing the floor surface [115].

Identification of Objects Handled by the Decedent before Death

Kodama and colleagues conducted a study in which they analyzed microbial communities in order to determine objects that had been manipulated by a deceased individual prior to their death. The researchers specifically examined cadaver skin microbiomes from the right palm, as well as 100 various objects (such as phones or lighters) that may have been handled by the victim, at 16 different crime scenes. Their findings revealed that post-mortem skin microbiomes remained relatively stable during transport and storage in the morgue. This data could potentially be utilized to estimate the post-mortem interval (PMI) and could facilitate the recovery of microorganisms directly from the cadaver, rather than solely at the scene of the crime. However, it remains challenging to determine the exact timeframe in which the victim had come into contact with these objects [79].

Utilizing Microbiome Analysis for Estimation of the Post-Mortem Interval (PMI)

Estimating postmortem interval (PMI) is a well-documented and widely recognized application of microbial community analysis. Determining PMI can be crucial in establishing the time of death or certifying deaths. However, estimating PMI is often challenging due to the intricate nature of death mechanisms. Following death, the body undergoes progressive and irreversible physical and chemical alterations. This decomposition of organic matter, notably cadaver decomposition, involves a variety of biological agents such as cell enzymes, bacteria, fungi, protozoa, insects, or scavengers, as well as non-biological elements influenced by the surrounding environment such as humidity and weather patterns. Insects, invertebrates, and other organic components all play various roles in the decomposition process, following a specific and organized sequence [116-118].

The Post-Mortem Interval (PMI) is traditionally determined by physical changes that occur after death, such as rigor mortis, lividity, body temperature, and activity in the upper gastrointestinal tract. Nevertheless, these changes occur early in the post-mortem process, providing only a rough estimate of the PMI. More recent methods for estimating the PMI include thanatochemistry, DNA/RNA degradation, and entomology. Factors like rain, cold temperatures, indoor settings (with limited or no insect presence), and seasonal variations can impede the study of insects and their behaviors. It is necessary to explore alternative approaches for estimating the PMI [117-119].

In recent times, there has been a growing interest in evaluating changes in microbial communities as a means of determining the post-mortem interval (PMI) and circumstances surrounding death. Metcalf *et al.* noted that microbial communities undergo distinct changes at different stages of cadaver decomposition, leading to the concept of a "microbial clock." The presence of bacteria in internal organs is closely associated with decomposition, with microbial cells accounting for 75-90% of all cells present before death. Two approaches are typically employed to study the evolution of microbiomes during decomposition: (i) the investigation of thanatomicrobiomes, which focuses on microorganisms found in internal organs and cavities following death; and (ii) the examination of epinecrotic communities, which involves the study of prokaryotes, protists, fungi, and eukaryotes residing on the surfaces of the deceased [120- 123].

The progression of microbial communities following a specific pattern is consistent and foreseeable within each individual. Commensal bacteria are involved in processing cellular byproducts that are produced when cells lyse due to oxygen deprivation and are recognized as a significant element in the breakdown of a corpse. Once deceased, internal bacteria commence the digestion of the body internally, while enzymes from dead cells deteriorate tissues. The reduction in biomass primarily occurs due to the activities of insects and microorganisms. The process of decomposition involves two distinct phases for bacterial communities [124, 125].

Various anaerobic organisms proliferate within the abdominal cavity during the initial 9-day post-mortem. These microbial processes contribute to the generation of gases within various body regions and the breakdown of tissues. Subsequently, the introduction of oxygen facilitates the growth of aerobic bacteria and opportunistic pathogens, specifically creating an environment conducive to the proliferation of Proteobacteria due to an increase in pH levels. As decomposition progresses, changes in environmental conditions disrupt the balance of normal bacterial flora, allowing opportunistic pathogens to establish and multiply. The microbial composition of the decaying body shifts to mirror the microbial communities in the vicinity. By analyzing the microbiomes of soil surrounding gravesites, the abdominal cavity, and skin, researchers can track the succession of specific bacteria to estimate the post-mortem interval (PMI). Metcalf and colleagues demonstrated a precise estimation of time since death, with an accuracy of approximately 3 days, by utilizing 16S and 18S rDNA analysis in combination. However, some variability among individuals in the progression of bacterial communities cannot be entirely ruled out [126-128].

A multitude of environmental factors, including temperature, soil composition, humidity levels, oxygen availability, precipitation patterns, and the presence of insects or scavenging animals, can affect the sequential breakdown of a microbiome. The decomposition of soil is intricately linked to microbial processes. Changes in soil chemistry, particularly in terms of organic carbon, ammonia, and nitrogen levels, occur during the process of cadaver decomposition. A study by Hyde *et al.* observed the decomposition of two similar cadavers over a roughly two-week period, one in September and the other in November. The environmental conditions surrounding the cadavers played a significant role in influencing the bacterial communities and decomposition progress. Variations were also detected in the microbial makeup and organization across different body sites. Guo *et al.* confirmed that various factors, such as the initial settlement of microbial communities on and within the cadaver, the cadaver's surroundings, and the sampling method employed, can impact outcomes. They discovered that the presence or absence of sarcosaprophagous insects had minimal effect on microbial community taxa, thus eliminating one environmental factor from consideration [122- 126].

The microbial clock is most precise within 48 hours of detection when the body is fresh and has not been contaminated by soil microorganisms. As time passes, the margin of error increases. In cases of advanced decomposition, the estimated post-mortem interval (PMI) can have an error rate of approximately 5-7 days. When only the skeleton remains, PMI can be determined by analyzing the microbes present in the bones. Various factors such as age, cause of death, underlying health conditions, drug use, and diet can affect the accuracy of PMI estimation and should be taken into account during calculation. Research by Pechal *et al.* revealed that factors like sex and organ type can significantly influence PMI determination, whereas variables like location, season of death, and weight do not have the same impact. The circumstances of death also appear to affect the diversity of bacteria recovered from the body: individuals who died from heart diseases had a lower bacterial diversity, while those who experienced violent deaths exhibited a more varied microbial composition [127].

Ultimately, the efficacy of proteomic methodologies has been scrutinized. While MALDI-ToF analysis has successfully identified a large portion of bacterial populations, notable instances of inaccurate results have been attributed to heightened peptide signals within muscular tissues, necessitating further advancements [126].

Utilization of Geolocation for Assessing and Identifying Soil Microbiomes

Microbial communities exhibit variation based on the specific locations from which samples are obtained. The bacterial makeup is influenced by factors such as climate, altitude, urban surroundings, and soil characteristics inherent to the area. The soil, being diverse, transportable, and a source of crucial geographical data, may have relevance in tracking human migration or the movement of a deceased individual. Nevertheless, certain constraints exist due to personal habits, travel history, or health conditions. Soil can adhere to various substrates and be collected for analysis. Its utility extends to determining the source of an unidentified specimen, narrowing down search areas, or comparing samples from a suspect with those from a crime scene. Chemical, mineral, and organic properties of soils have been traditionally studied, including their type, color, size, and composition. Assessments can encompass palynology, focusing on pollen grains and spores to establish a unique pollen profile associated with a specific location. While these methodologies may lack adequate specificity at present, their integration with investigations of microbial communities could enhance effectiveness [128, 129]

Soil harbours a multitude of microorganisms that coexist and interact with each other, contributing to a distinct characteristic of the area under investigation. The microbial populations in soil exhibit diverse compositions across different soil types, primarily influenced by factors such as organic or mineral content, soil pH, alkalinity, and environmental variations. In the MiSAFE initiative, Demanèche and colleagues compared two metagenomic methodologies for forensic applications. By analyzing a simulated crime scene where drugs were concealed beneath disturbed soil, significant differences were observed between two scenarios – one in close proximity to the crime scene (approximately 25 meters) and another located about 1 kilometer away from the suspect's residence. This research illustrated the ability to identify variations between soils through taxonomic and functional analyses, facilitating the linkage or exclusion of sites based on distinct bacterial communities present [128].

Habtom and colleagues conducted an assessment on the importance of identifying soil origin based on microbial communities. They collected samples from five established research sites located 260 km apart in Israel, each site consisting of two to four different types of soil. Their findings indicated that microbial communities within the same site demonstrated greater similarity compared to communities from the same soil type in different locations. Moreover, a notable correlation was identified between the geographical distance separating soil samples and the microbial communities present. Nevertheless, notable variations were observed in bacterial communities among the different soil types within each location [128].

Factors that impact the analysis of microbiome

Dobay and colleagues conducted an assessment of the evolution of microbiomes in samples collected from various body locations and fluids (such as saliva, vaginal fluid, skin, menstrual and peripheral blood, and semen) maintained at room temperature for a period of 30 days. They noted that the composition of microorganisms present was unique to the specific body site. Exposure to environmental conditions did not lead to noteworthy changes in these microbial communities, as each body location retained its characteristic microbial profile. Diez Lopez and associates examined additional factors including variations in sample substrate, storage methods, and environmental conditions (such as temperature or humidity levels, and sample freshness), all of which demonstrated consistent microbiome findings [130].

The impact of different storage durations and temperatures on the microbiome found on the scalp and pubic hairs was investigated. In a study conducted by Williams and colleagues, various storage temperatures commonly used in forensic laboratories - room temperature, +4 °C, and −20 °C - were evaluated over a period of 6 weeks. It was found that neither the duration nor the temperature of storage significantly affected the composition of microbial communities [131].

Song *et al.* conducted a study to assess how various conservation methods affect the faecal microbiome. They examined the effects of immediate extraction versus storage at different temperatures (ranging from -20°C to room temperature), as well as the use of a preservative. The results showed that storage temperature did not have a significant impact on the faecal microbiome. However, immediate freezing with the addition of a preservative (such as ethanol) demonstrated the least disturbance to the composition and diversity of bacterial communities [72].

Sampling and Lab Protocol

Hannsen and colleagues conducted a study on the potential impact of sampling and laboratory procedures on the detection and identification of saliva deposited on human skin. They evaluated three different sampling techniques: cotton swabs, synthetic swabs, and tape. The samples used in the study included pure saliva from the mouth, saliva deposited between fingers, and samples recovered directly from the fingers. The study found that cotton swabs, which are commonly used in forensic investigations, were less effective at recovering saliva compared to synthetic swabs and tape. The bacterial communities found in saliva from the mouth were more concentrated than those recovered from the skin. Additionally, using tape for recovery resulted in greater bacterial diversity. Skin samples also exhibited more bacterial variation compared to saliva samples. The study also found that oral, vaginal, and faecal samples could be easily distinguished, while nasal samples were often mistaken for skin samples [133].

Saliva samples adhering to the skin in conjunction with the skin microbiome can complicate interpretation. Variations in individuals were noted as a result of lifestyle or health factors, rather than the sampling method itself. Various other factors, including the extraction method, sampling location on the body, and library preparation steps, may also impact the findings. It is essential to utilize standardized sampling techniques and protocols [67].

Despite the fact that the sampling technique did not directly influence the analysis, its significance in the abundance of retrieved microbial communities was assessed. A comparison was made among four different sampling methods employed to assess the skin microbiome (swabbing, scraping, glove juice sampling, and punch biopsy). Among these methods, glove juice was identified as the most effective due to its ability to detect bacteria located in the deeper layers of the skin using a less invasive approach compared to biopsy. Additionally, glove juice sampling was found to be more reliable over time in comparison to swabbing, which recovered a higher number of pathogens but was prone to higher levels of contamination [134].

The duration between the deposit and collection of samples is crucial as it may pose challenges in accurately identifying unique microbial communities. This is due to the fact that samples taken at a specific time may not necessarily reflect the initial microbiota [135].

Chase *et al.* emphasized the impact of sequencing runs on result quality. Variations in microbial composition were documented across runs, likely attributable to low-abundance taxa. Consequently, the effectiveness of sampling, its redundancy, and utilization of technical replicates contribute to result quality enhancement [136].

Influence of Hand Washing

Tims *et al.* conducted a study comparing microbial populations pre- and post-hand washing with hospital soap and air drying. Although there were variations among participants, the cutaneous microbiome remained relatively consistent after washing. The potential for contamination was evident through the transfer of microbes from the environment. Interestingly, the analysis of cutaneous samples from diverse countries revealed minimal influence of geographical locations on microbial communities. In contrast, Fierer *et al.* found conflicting results regarding the effect of hand washing on microbial composition. It was observed that the predominant taxa, including the core microbiome, were consistently present before and after washing, however, the timing between washing and sampling impacted the composition and any changes. Diez Lopez *et al.* noted that wearing gloves prior to sampling did not significantly affect microbial detection. While the study did not investigate the use of cosmetic products, it was suggested that antibiotic use did not have a substantial impact on the variability of hand microbiomes [137].

Environmental Conditions

Assessment of the influence of geographic location, seasonal fluctuations, and indoor environments revealed a continuous interaction between human and environmental microbiomes. A study was conducted to identify the origins of variability by examining samples from various offices in three distinct cities over a period of six weeks. It was observed that the specific location within the office had an effect on the microbial makeup and richness (with floor samples displaying higher diversity), while the type of surface material did not have a significant impact. Consistent with previous findings, the microbiomes in each city displayed unique characteristics. The microbial composition of the offices was naturally shaped by human interactions, particularly through the skin microbiome [136].

A research study carried out in domestic kitchens revealed the frequent exposure to a variety of bacteria species from both humans and food items. This finding presents a unique perspective in forensics as it suggests that a person can leave behind evidence of their presence in a space through their bacterial profile. In contrast, it also shows that any surface tested and studied could potentially be tainted by an external bacterial origin. Therefore, it is crucial to select the appropriate surfaces to test for forensic purposes meticulously [138].

Research conducted on household surfaces revealed that the predominant bacteria found were closely associated with the occupants of the homes. The microbiota consisted mainly of skin-related species from areas such as the nose, hands, and feet, as well as microorganisms from the surrounding environment. These microbial communities were consistent and distinct for each household. However, the accuracy of the findings declined over time, indicating that the microbiota deteriorated after being deposited on a surface, without any external interference. This decline in results quality was hastened in public spaces experiencing frequent alterations compared to a private residence [139].

The diversity of the microbiota was found to increase with certain lifestyle factors, such as living with pets. A study was conducted to examine the impact of children and pets on the microbial composition within households. It was observed that family members shared a significant level of bacterial diversity, except for very young children who had a distinct microbiota. Furthermore, the microbial communities of humans were found to bear similarities to those of their canine companions, with a notable exchange of microorganisms occurring between the hand microbiota of individuals and their dogs. Interestingly, the microbiota of individuals living with other types of pets did not appear to have a substantial influence [140].

Microbiota and Real Cases

Microbiome studies in real forensic sciences with legal implications have been sparsely documented, largely due to the need for further development and adaptation of Next-Generation Sequencing (NGS) technology for forensic applications, as well as limited routine use of this technology by forensic teams. The integration of microbiome studies with human genetic approaches remains an area requiring clarification.

Quaak *et al.* reported on two cases involving the application of microbiome studies in forensic investigations. In the first case, the detection of an unknown male genetic profile in stained tissue near a car used in a house robbery led to the apprehension of a suspect with a matching genetic profile. Despite the defense's claim that the genetic profile could have originated from an unrelated activity, a microbial analysis linking the genetic profile to faecal samples ultimately resulted in the suspect's conviction [141].

The second case involved a sexual assault perpetrated by a nurse at a hospital, which included both anal and vaginal assault. Analysis of bacterial populations in samples obtained from the accused's genital area revealed a combination of faecal and vaginal microbiota present in both the victims and the perpetrator, leading to a conviction in court [141].

An additional investigation involved a case of a minor being raped. A potential object linked to the sexual assault was confiscated. The genetic samples obtained comprised a blend of DNA from the perpetrator and the victim. Analysis of the microbes indicated a significant presence of vaginal bacterial flora on the object employed during the rape. Furthermore, another instance showcasing the application of microbiome in forensic investigations pertained to a scenario of rape through digital penetration. Analysis of a swab extracted from the suspect's finger revealed a combination of the suspect's DNA and the victim's DNA. The predominant microbial community identified was characterized by vaginal microbiota, providing evidence of digital penetration [142].

Potential Bacterial biomarkers for insect colonization in Forensic Cases

The utilization of entomology in the realm of forensic sciences for estimating the postmortem interval (PMI) has been firmly established for many years, relying on the presence and behavior of necrophagous insects in decomposed human remains. In recent times, there has been a growing interest in researching the microbiome of necrophagous insects, with the aim of understanding the relationship between bacteria and various insect species. Currently, a significant proportion of studies on insect microbiomes have primarily examined issues such as antimicrobial resistance and disease transmission [143- 157].

Only a limited number of research studies have explored the bacterial makeup and microbiome metagenomic evaluation across various necrophagous insect species, with the aim of providing valuable information applicable to the realm of forensic sciences. To the best of the researchers' knowledge, no studies have specifically delved into the amplification and quantification of *Wohlfahrtiimonas chitiniclastica* (*W. chitiniclastica*) and *Ignatzschineria indica* transmission from the immature stages of *Lucilia illustris Meigen*, 1826 (Diptera: Calliphoridae) to the colonized tissues. These two bacterial species, which are Gram-negative and aerobic, are classified under the Proteobacteria phylum and Xanthomonadaceae family and were initially identified and described in association with necrophagous insect species. While *W. chitiniclastica* was initially isolated and characterized in the flesh fly *Wohlfahrtia magnifica* (Schiner, 1862) (Diptera: Sarcophagidae), I. indica was first discovered in adult flesh flies. These bacterial strains have also been identified in hospital cases involving sepsis, bacteremia, and myiasis, underscoring their significance in certain clinical scenarios [156- 164]

Under certain circumstances or during postmortem examinations, human remains may lack insect eggs, larvae, and/or adults, or they may simply go unnoticed. Understanding how insect-specific bacteria are transferred could provide valuable evidence of necrophagous insect species having been present on the decomposing body, potentially from the early stages of colonization. This can be achieved by conducting a quantitative analysis of the bacterial content, which, as demonstrated in this study, varies based on the insect's developmental stage and/or the tissue it has consumed. By examining changes in bacterial quantity throughout different insect developmental stages and linking these variations to the time of colonization, insect-associated bacterial species could potentially serve as post-mortem interval (PMI) biomarkers in the future [165].

The main goal of the current research was to quantitatively investigate two specific bacterial taxa found in insects at various stages of development (egg, first, second, and third instar larvae) and analyze the transfer of these bacteria to the feeding substrate based on larval stages. This study offers initial findings on quantifying bacterial transfer, which could have significant implications in the field of forensic sciences. Additionally, the importance of this study stems from the fact that these bacterial taxa were identified in various necrophagous insect species from different geographic locations, making the data valuable to the international scientific community as potential indicators of postmortem interval in the absence of insects. However, further studies are required before definitive conclusions can be made, including the investigation of other insect-specific bacteria and species that inhabit decomposed remains [166- 168].

Lucilia illustris Meigen (*L. illustris*), 1826 (Diptera: Calliphoridae) was chosen for the study due to its synanthropic environmental presence and abundant population during the summer months, making it one of the first insects to colonize carrion. Adult *L. illustris* specimens were gathered on three separate occasions (approximately 30 specimens per sampling) from an urban area in Bucharest, Romania (N44°26′49.349′ E26°2′45.352″) in July 2017 [165].

The adult insects, captured using entomological nets, were placed in sterilized rearing chambers alongside beef or pork liver tissues, maintaining consistent laboratory conditions (25 °C ± 1 and 60% relative humidity, LD 12:12). Following oviposition, the eggs of *L. illustris* were transferred to small, sterile rearing jars measuring 21× 12 cm in diameter (BioQuip Products, Rancho Dominguez, CA, USA), where the immature stages were raised under identical laboratory conditions with daily sampling, in the presence of 375 g of liver. Control-rearing jars without colonization were also set up, containing equal amounts of pork or beef liver and maintained under the same sterile experimental conditions (Figure 4) [166].

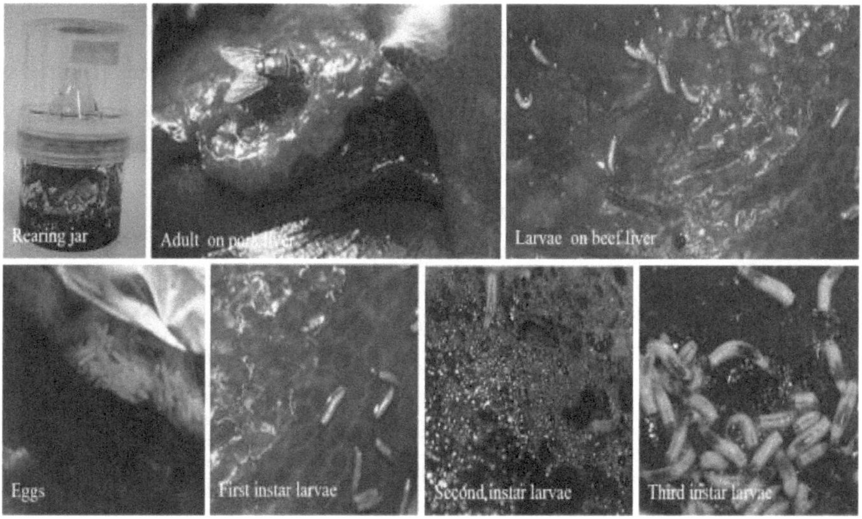

Figure 4: a laboratory arrangement designed for studying the developmental stages of *Lucilia illustris* using beef and pork liver as food sources [166]

Bacterial-specific *gyr*B primers

Due to the significant resemblance in the 16S rRNA genes of the studied species, with an 82.6% similarity rate, individual primer pairs were developed for each bacterial species using fragments of the DNA gyrase subunit B gene (*gyr*B). The resulting amplicon length encompassed 140 bp for *W. chitiniclastica* and 262 bp for *Ignatzschineria indica* (*I. indica*). Both the PCR amplification (as shown in Fig. 5a) and the melting temperature curves (as depicted in Fig. 5b) demonstrated a high level of specificity in amplifying the genes corresponding to *W. chitiniclastica* and *I. indica* [167] .

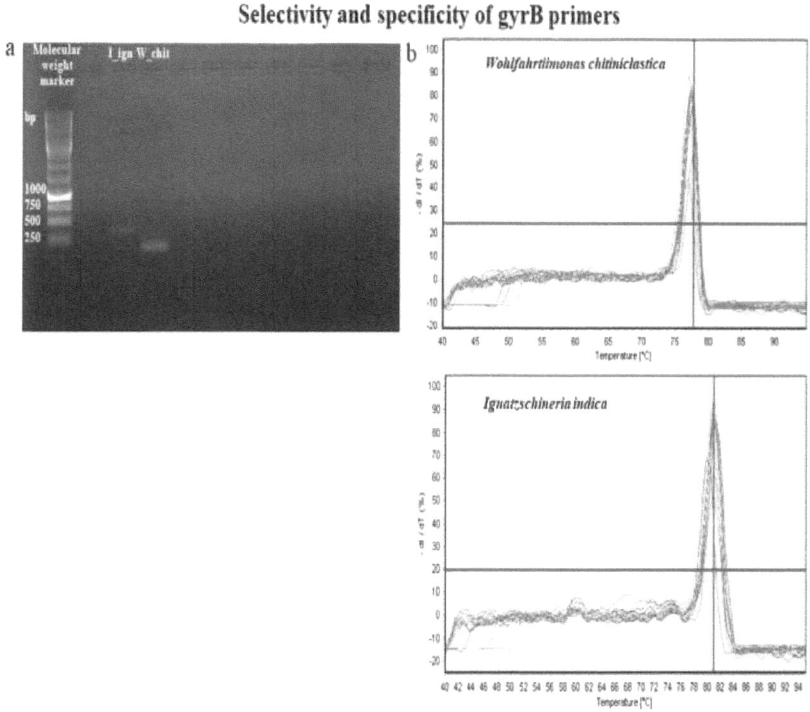

Figure 5: PCR amplification was conducted on gene fragments of *Wohlfahrtiimonas chitiniclastica* and Ignatzschineria indica *gyr*B. The resulting products included bacterial gyrB amplicons and the melting temperatures of the amplified gene fragments from both bacterial species were determined[167]

***Wohlfahrtiimonas chitiniclastica* in insect immature stages**

Wohlfahrtiimonas chitiniclastica was found across all stages of development of *L. illustris*, beginning with the initial immature stage, the egg (illustrated in Figure 6). The abundance of *W. chitiniclastica* in egg samples collected from the pork liver feeding substrate was lower at 101.68, compared to a significantly higher bacterial content observed in first instar larvae samples, which was approximately 103 times greater than in the egg samples. In contrast, *W. chitiniclastica* maintained consistent levels across the three larval stages, with comparable amounts recorded at 105.09, 105.02, and 104.60 respectively [168].

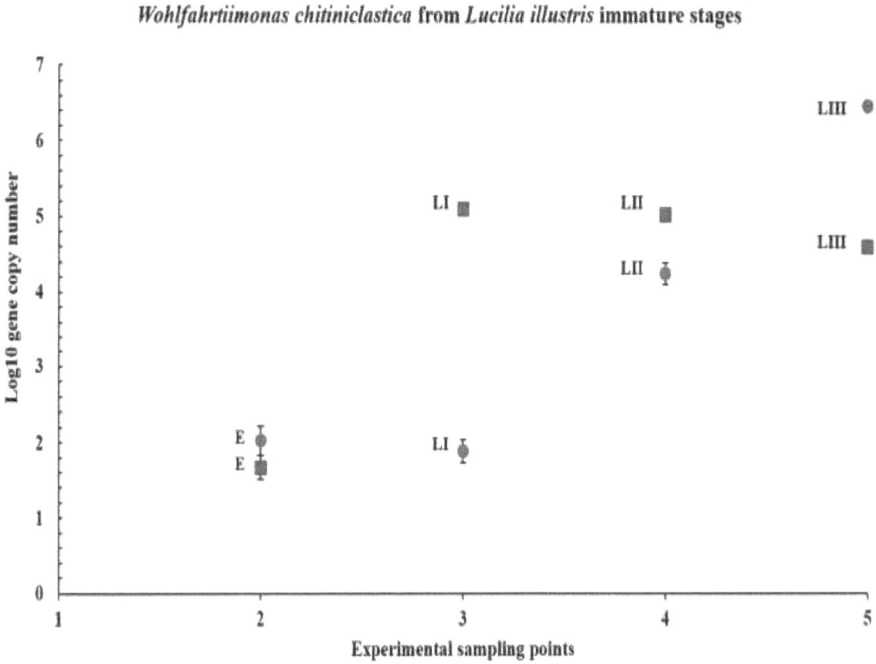

Figure 6: The prevalence of *Wohlfahrtiimonas chitiniclastica* was measured in various developmental stages of *Lucilia illustris* (including eggs and first, second, and third instar larvae) raised on diets of pork and beef liver. Error bars represent standard deviations [168]

A reduced bacterial transfer rate was observed in the first and second instar larvae when the substrate was beef liver, while the egg and first instar larvae samples showed similar levels of abundance. Additionally, the highest abundances of *W. chitiniclastica* were found in the second and third larval stages [169].

In comparison to immature stages that consumed a diet of pork liver and exhibited a consistent trend following initial quantitative growth of *W. chitiniclastica* in the first instar larvae, immature stages that were fed beef liver displayed an increasing bacterial dynamic trend, despite lower quantities in the first two instars. These variations in bacterial quantities of *W. chitiniclastica* from specimens reared on pork versus beef could be attributed to differences in the feeding substrate [170].

Ignatzschineria indica in insect immature stages

In the instance of *I. indica*, the density of bacterial cells appeared to vary depending on the type of tissue used as a food source. When pork tissue was used as the substrate, *I. indica* was detected in all stages of immature *L. illustris*, with minimal presence in egg samples (102.2), peaking in the third instar larvae (106.1). This marked a 102.72-fold increase compared to the egg samples, demonstrating an increasing trend during larval growth [171].

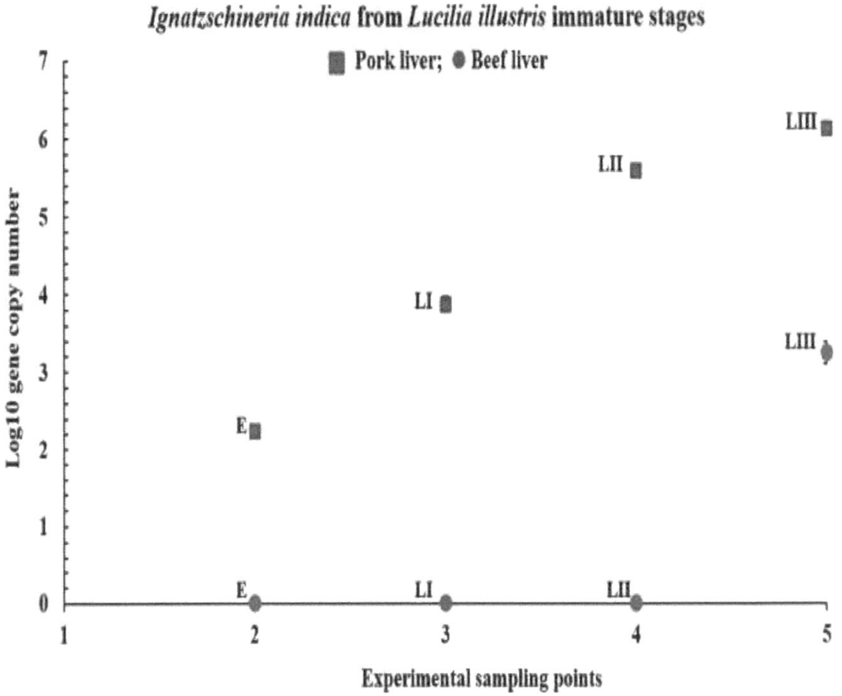

Figure 7: The prevalence of *Ignatzschineria indica* was measured in the immature stages of *Lucilia illustris* (Egg, first instar larvae, second instar larvae, third instar larvae) that were fed with pork and beef liver. Error bars were used to represent the standard deviations [171].

Alternatively, *I. indica* was only detectable in the third instar larvae (103.2) when identified in the immature stages of insects raised on a beef liver diet, showing a decrease of 10−1.89× compared to larvae fed with pork liver. The presence of *I. indica* was not evident in the earlier stages of insect development due to its very limited quantities, ultimately representing a 50% lower abundance than in insect specimens fed with pork liver **[172]**.

Pork and beef liver tissues

In the scenario involving the pork liver substrate, both *W. chitiniclastica* and *I. indica* exhibited transfer after three days of experimentation, displaying a consistent trend on days 3 and 4 with a ratio of 105.1–105.3. The bacterial content of *I. indica* surpassed that of *W. chitiniclastica* by 102.47 times on day 5. The elevated bacterial levels detected in the pork liver sample on day 5 were predominantly attributed to *I. indica*, reaching 106.4 **[173]**.

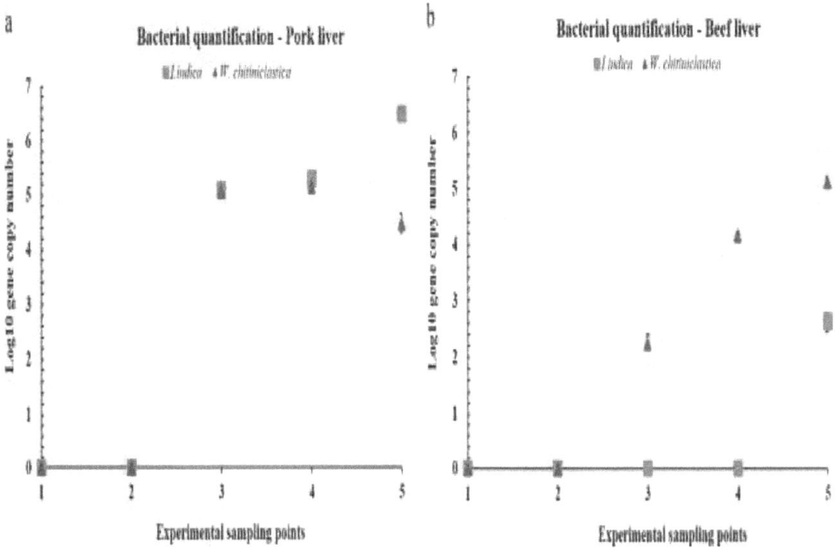

Figure 8: The prevalence of *I. indica* and *W. chitiniclastica* was observed in both pork liver and beef liver samples. Error bars were used to represent the standard deviations [173]

Wohlfahrtiimonas chitiniclastica was detected in the beef liver on day 3 and continued to increase steadily until day 5, reaching similar levels to those found in pork liver. There was no presence of *I. indica* in the beef-feeding substrate during the initial four days of the experiment, which aligns with the early developmental stages of *L. illustris* larvae. *I. indica* was only observed on day 5, with a significantly lower abundance compared to *W. chitiniclastica*. While the abundance of bacteria varied between pork and beef-feeding substrates, the highest levels for both bacterial taxa were found in insect specimens raised on pork liver. Initially, the bacterial content of both taxa was undetectable in the liver samples and reference liver used in the study. The process of carcass decomposition, whether human or animal, depends on various factors such as the cause of death, post-mortem conditions, geographic location, weather conditions, and specific environmental circumstances. Decomposition typically begins soon after vital signs cease, leading to biochemical changes and bacterial proliferation from the gastrointestinal tract. These changes attract a range of necrophagous insect species that colonize the cadaver in a specific sequence over time. In warmer temperatures, decomposing bodies attract Diptera and Coleoptera species more rapidly, which feed on the remains and reproduce. Upon colonization of the carcass by necrophagous insects, there is also a transfer of microbiome from the insects to the remains [176].

The activity periods, colonization patterns, and feeding preferences of insect species have been extensively studied. Yet, there is still much to learn about the transfer of specific bacterial species among insects during their developmental cycle and their transfer to colonized tissues and substrates. Previous research on characterizing bacterial diversity in various insect species has utilized traditional microbiological cultivation methods as well as modern molecular high throughput 16S rRNA gene sequencing techniques [185]. Due to their significant roles in the fields of medicine, veterinary science, and forensics, muscids and calliphorids have been employed in research on the microbiome composition of insects, with a particular emphasis on the transmission of pathogens and the presence of antimicrobial resistance. Additionally, research has been conducted on the bacterial communities present in these insects, exploring their interactions and functions throughout various stages of insect development [186].

"In this context, *Musca domestica Linnaeus*, 1758 (Diptera: Muscidae) has frequently been utilized as a model organism in scientific studies due to its close association with human habitats and its ability to easily transmit various pathogens. The primary focus of the research has been on characterizing the bacterial diversity and identifying bacterial pathogens present in this species of fly. Additionally, other insect species, such as *Wohlfahrtia magnifica* (Schiner, 1862) (Diptera: Sarcophagidae), have been studied to assess their bacterial composition. Tóth and colleagues conducted a study on the bacteria associated with *W. magnifica* due to its potential to cause myiasis in domestic animals, particularly in Eurasia. Their research highlighted the likely presence of Ignatzschineria species in the foregut of the insect larvae. Both *Ignatzschineria* and *Wohlfahrtiimonas* were found to exhibit significant chitinase activity, potentially playing a crucial role in the developmental stage of the flies. While Tóth and collaborators did not conduct a quantitative analysis, they identified both bacterial species in the larval stages of *W. magnifica*. In the experiment, not only were these bacterial species identified, but their quantitative abundance was also assessed, revealing that these microbes are specific to insects and that a detailed examination of them could enhance understanding of their role as biomarkers for insect colonization [188].

Moreover, Zheng and colleagues conducted an extensive examination of the bacterial diversity found in various life stages of the black soldier fly, *Hermetia illucens* (Linnaeus, 1758) (Diptera: Stratiomyidae). Their primary aim was to investigate the transmission of pathogens during *H. illucens'* developmental cycle. Despite this focus, the analysis of bacterial diversity unveiled the presence of *Ignatzschineria* spp. in the specimens studied. This finding further supports the established association of this bacteria with fly species from different Diptera families [188].

In a separate study, Weatherbee and team explored the microbiome of larvae masses from different *Calliphoridae* species (Phormia regina Meigen, 1826, *Lucilia coeruleiviridis* Macquart, 1855, *Cochliomyia macellaria* (Fabricius, 1775) and identified Xanthomonadaceae as a predominant family. However, they did not provide taxonomic categorizations beyond the family level. Nevertheless, their research demonstrated an increase in Xanthomonadaceae levels during the decomposition process. These findings mirror the observations regarding the temporal patterns of bacterial taxa abundance during both the insect larval stages and liver colonization [178].

A recent research study focused on investigating the bacterial diversity present in the third instar larvae of the stable fly *Stomoxys calcitrans* (Linnaeus, 1758) (Diptera: Muscidae). The findings revealed *Ignatzschineria* as one of the most abundant bacterial genera in the larvae samples. Interestingly, *Ignatzschineria* showed higher prevalence in the fly larvae samples compared to the surrounding living substrates, mirroring previous findings in which *I. indica* dominated in *L. illustris* immature stages. Furthermore, the microbiome of other synanthropic species, such as the oriental latrine fly *Chrysomya megacephala* (Fabricius, 1794), was also analyzed during its developmental cycle for comparison [185].

In the course of the respective investigation, both *Ignatzschineria* and *Wohlfahrtiimonas* were detected in the insect specimens, although these genera were not found among the predominant gut bacteria as observed in previous experiments. Nevertheless, the presence of these bacteria in various Diptera species underscores their potential utility as universal indicators for estimating the time of insect colonization [185].

In another research endeavor focusing on the persistence of antibiotic-resistant bacteria carried out by Wei and colleagues, *Ignatzschineria* and *Wohlfahrtiimonas* were identified in experiments involving *Proteus mirabilis* (*P. mirabilis*) with *Musca domestica* (*M. domestica*) and *Lucilia sericata* (*L. sericata*). The researchers utilized quantitative PCR assays to track *P. mirabilis* levels and duration of survival in the flies' digestive system, as well as employing 454 pyrosequencing to analyze the entire microbiome. qPCR was utilized here as an investigative method, albeit focusing on a different bacterial taxonomy. Notably, the microbiome analysis through 454 pyrosequencing uncovered the presence of *Wohlfahrtiimonas* in *L. sericata* samples. Additionally, *Ignatzschineria* was recognized as a dominant bacterium in green bottle flies collected during the summer months, aligning with other identification of *Ignatzschineria indica* in *L. illustris* specimens [188].

Wohlfahrtiimonas chitiniclastica was determined to be a prevalent bacterial taxon in both culture isolates and clone library samples during the study conducted by Gupta and colleagues, with *Ignatzschineria* spp. also being identified in the survey. Both *Ignatzschineria* and *Wohlfahrtiimonas* were also detected in another investigation by Gupta and colleagues, analyzing the bacterial composition in the intestinal gut of adult sarcophagids. In addition, these taxa were found to be common among the cultured bacteria identified in samples from both flesh flies' adults and larvae, although *Ignatzschineria* was more frequently observed in both culture and clone sequences [188].

While most studies conducted thus far have primarily focused on bacteria associated with muscids, research has also been extended to include green flies. Singh and collaborators examined the bacterial content in *Lucilia sericata* and Lucilia cuprina species (Diptera: Calliphoridae), highlighting horizontal transmission of bacteria as more prevalent than trans-generational inheritance. Although taxonomic identification only extended to the genus level in their experiment, *Ignatzschineria* was one of the top five dominant genera found in both insect species, with no mention of *Wohlfahrtiimonas*. The authors noted a scarcity of data on bacteria associated with *Lucilia* species, with limited comprehensive investigations conducted on bacteria linked to green bottleflies. The current study introduces novel and preliminary findings on *W. chitiniclastica* and *I. indica*, aiming to contribute to expanding research in forensic entomology focused on necrophagous insect-associated bacterial communities [189].

Previous research studies have demonstrated the frequent presence and association of *Ignatzschineria* and *Wohlfahrtiimonas* with diverse insect species. The detection and quantification of these bacterial genera in necrophagous insects can offer insights into body colonization, even in the absence of adult or immature stages. This scenario may occur during crime scene investigations or autopsies when insect evidence is disregarded, particularly in the early stages of insect colonization. Nonetheless, this information could be utilized regardless of the presence or absence of entomological evidence to furnish additional data on the timing of colonization through bacterial quantification. In this particular study, both *Ignatzschineria* and *Wohlfahrtiimonas* were identified in insects and liver tissue samples, exhibiting similar levels in pork liver samples. This suggests that they could serve as potential bacterial indicators for insect colonization, aligning with the core hypothesis of the experiment [189]. Although further research is necessary to validate the role of these bacterial species as colonization markers under varying conditions and substrates, this study marks the first recognition of the forensic utility of *Ignatzschineria* and *Wohlfahrtiimonas* [190].

Isolation and identification of virulent bacteria from forensic flies

Forensic entomology examines the ecological and biological characteristics of arthropod populations that inhabit new rhizosphere environments. This field is closely associated with forensic investigation. When vertebrate scavengers are absent, animal remains attract a diverse array of insects that work with anaerobes to accelerate the decomposition process. Flies are typically the first insects to colonize a deceased body. The specific species of flies involved may vary depending on the location, but numerous studies have indicated that the main species belong to a limited number of families, including Calliphoridae, Sarcophagidae, and Muscidae [189- 202].

Bacteria play a crucial role in various stages of decomposition, such as fresh, bloat, activity, advanced skeletonization, and skeletonization, influencing insect behavior to favor beneficial species and ward off harmful ones. Factors such as temperature, wind, moisture, geographical location, fauna composition, succession sequence, and the duration of insect presence all contribute to the decomposition process. Utilizing local climatic information and understanding the impact of native fauna can assist in estimating the postmortem interval (PMI). [203- 206].

Understanding the roles of microorganisms in the decomposition of carrion and their relevance to the estimation of post-mortem interval necessitates an appreciation of the fact that bacteria play a pivotal role as decomposers. Research by Janaway *et al.* [197] indicates that autolysis and bacterial activity in the tissues are key factors contributing to the initial breakdown of tissues. The proliferation of internal bacteria, such as those originating from the gastrointestinal (GI) tract, occurs as the tissues undergo decomposition. The transition from aerobic to anaerobic organisms is likely triggered by the depletion of oxygenated blood and subsequent loss of redox potential in the tissue. Flies have been identified as carriers of numerous bacterial, viral, and parasitic infections, with over 130 pathogens being transmitted by them. In healthcare settings and food establishments, flies have been observed carrying highly pathogenic bacteria. Among the most commonly transmitted pathogenic bacteria by flies are *Klebsiella* spp., *Salmonella*, *Pseudomonas aeruginosa*, *Campylobacter jejuni*, and *Edwardsiella* spp.. Furthermore, studies have shown that houseflies have the capacity to acquire and retain the contagious SARS-CoV-2 virus for up to 24 hours after exposure, enabling them to mechanically spread SARS-CoV-2 genomic RNA in the surrounding environment [198- 206].

The initial phase of decomposition in rabbit carcasses began with death and lasted for 12 hours postmortem. The bloated stage commenced on the first day after death and continued until the second day. The transition from the bloated stage to the active decay stage signaled the onset of liquefaction, which was confirmed by the presence of evidence of liquefaction on the fourth day following death. Advanced decay set in on the fourth day as the flesh of the rabbit carcass decomposed, starting from the head, limbs, and anus. The final stage of decomposition, known as the dry stage, was reached on the seventh day and persisted until the tenth day, during which time little odor was emitted and the bones became dry and hardened (refer to plate 1) [206].

The succession of forensic flies on a rabbit carcass

Some studies found that a total of 340 mature insects from 3 orders, 7 families, and 9 species were gathered during the various decomposition stages of a rabbit carcass. Initially, only 3 species of Diptera were found near the fresh carcass, with 2 *Chrysomya albiceps* flies, 2 *Musca domestica* flies, and 3 *Wohlfartia magnifica* flies being identified at the second decaying phase. As decomposition progressed, additional insect orders were attracted to the site, including 46 *Chrysomya albiceps*, 2 *Chrysomya megacephala*, 25 *Musca domestica*, 2 *Sarcophaga carnaria*, 23 *Wohlfartia magnifica*, and 6 Piophila casei flies [207].

During the decay stage, 2 species of Calliphoridae were collected, specifically 39 *Chrysomya albiceps* and 1 *Calliphora* sp.. Additionally, the family Sarcophagidae was represented by 7 *Wohlfartia magnifica* flies, while the family Muscidae had 41 *Musca domestica* specimens. Furthermore, 8 *Piophila casei* flies from the Piophilidae family were recorded. The dry stage of rabbit decomposition featured 11 *Chrysomya albiceps* flies, 11 *Musca domestica* flies, and beetles from the Histeridae and Dermestidae families, with 4 and 17 individuals captured, respectively. Finally, 90 ants belonging to the Hymenoptera order and Formicidae family were present at various stages of decomposition following the fresh stage [207].

Isolation of bacteria

A variety of media including Plate count agar (PCA), Eosin methylene blue (EMB), MacConkey agar (MAC), and Baird Parker (BP) were utilized for the purpose of isolating bacteria. The results of the research indicated that flies collected from different stages of decomposition of a rabbit carcass, ranging from fresh to decayed, were contaminated with varying levels of bacterial counts. Both Gram-positive and Gram-negative bacteria were isolated from the external surface of *Chrysomya albiceps* flies at all decomposition stages using the specified media (PCA, EMB, MAC, and BP) (Figure 9) [209].

https://journals.ekb.eg/article_358892_b9e32db23636f48767f03d967f1ef849.pdf

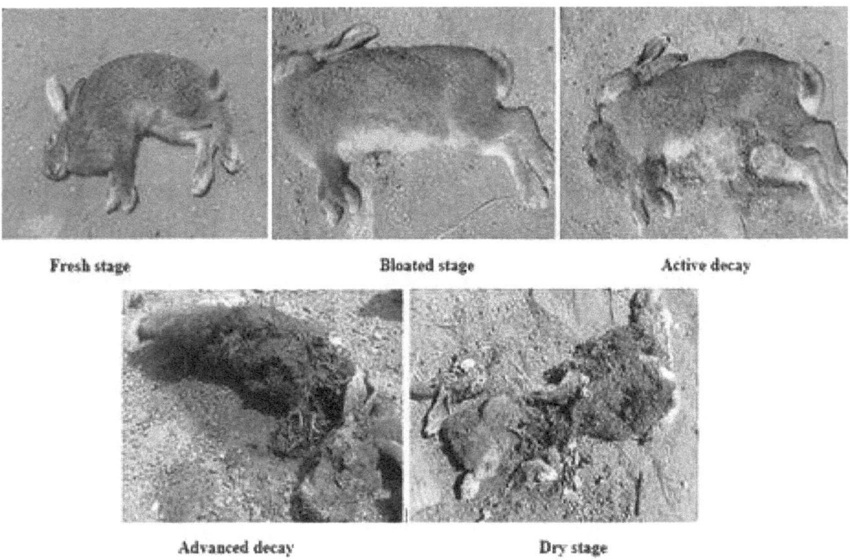

Figure 9: Decomposition stages of rabbit carcass [208]

Furthermore, it was evident that *Chrysomya megacephala* was observed only in the bloated stage. The identified bacteria were classified as Enterobacteriaceae and *Staphylococcus*. Conversely, *Calliphora* sp. was only found in the decay stage, with all isolated bacteria being Gram-negative Enterobacterales. Notably, *Musca domestica* flies were present at all stages of rabbit decomposition. The analysis revealed that *Musca domestica*, out of the over 340 flies examined, was the fly with the highest bacterial contamination. Interestingly, *Sarcophaga carnaria* flies were only found in the bloated stage, with the predominant bacterial isolates from the external surface being Gram-negative bacteria. Regarding the presence of *Wohlfartia magnifica*, it was noted in the initial three stages of decomposition. It was identified as the fly with the highest level of bacterial contamination among the 340 flies analyzed. *Piophila casei* was absent in the fresh stage but detected in both the bloated and decay stages. In the bloated stage, only Gram-positive Staphylococci were identified, while in the decay stage, Gram-positive and Gram-negative isolates were obtained (Figures 10, 11, 12, 13, 14, 15, 16, 17, 18, 19, 20, 21, 22) [209].

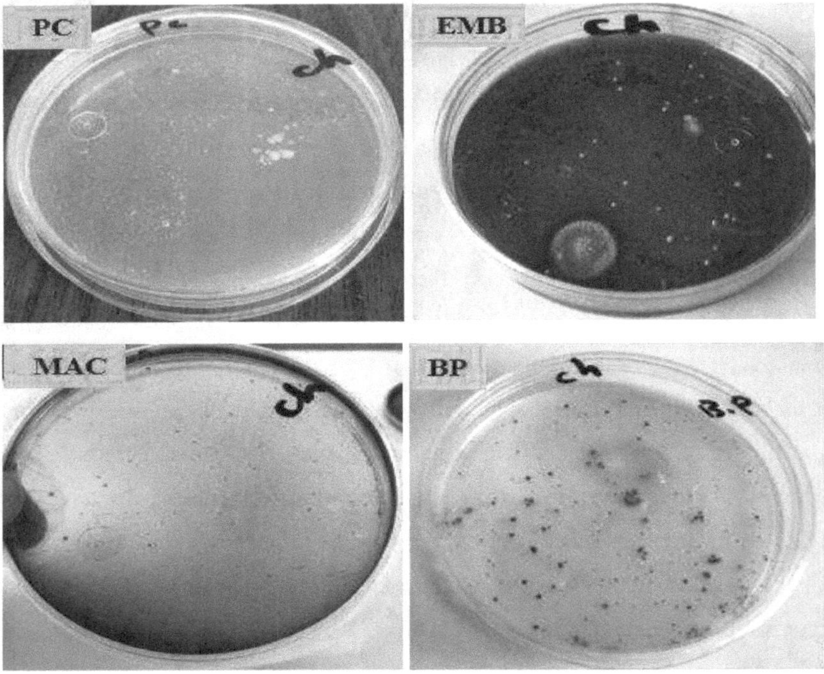

Figure 10: different bacterial colonies isolated from *Chrysomya albiceps* during the fresh stage [209]

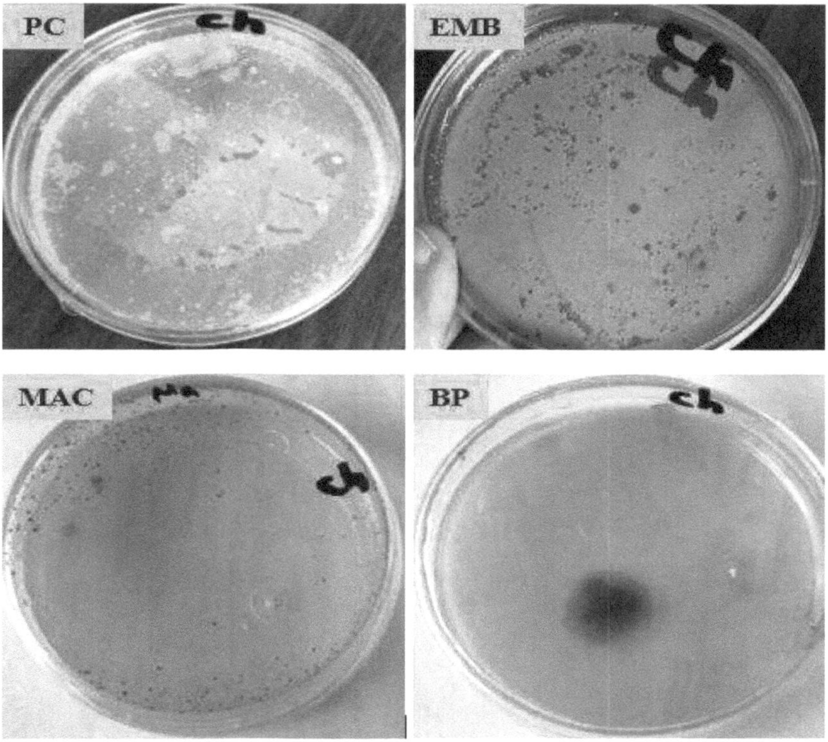

Figure 11: Different bacterial colonies isolated from *Chrysomya albiceps* during the bloated stage [209]

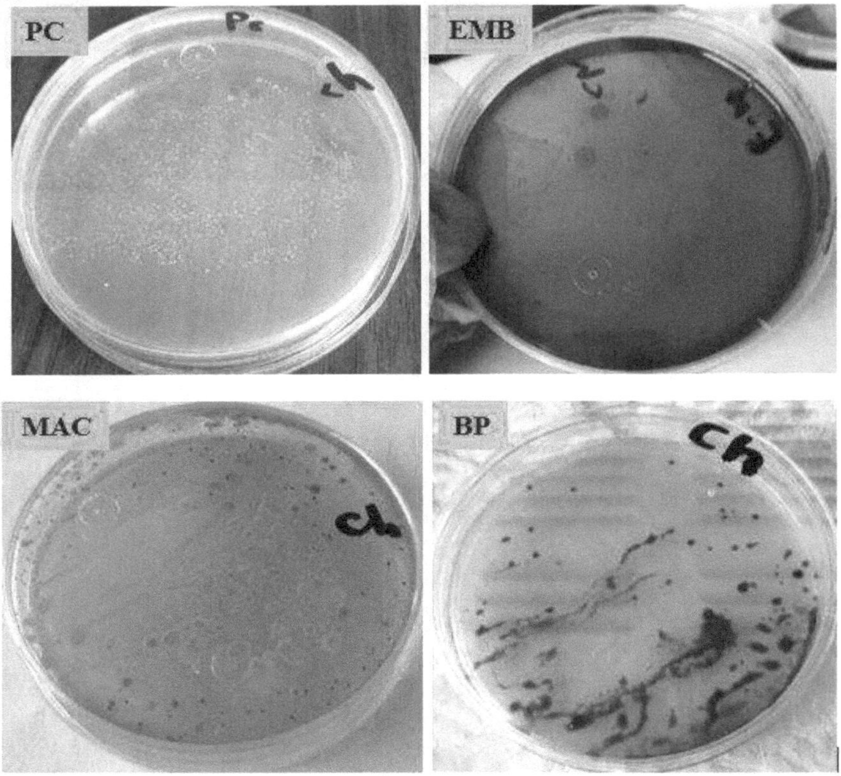

Figure 12: Different bacterial colonies isolated from *Chrysomya albiceps* during the decay stage [209]

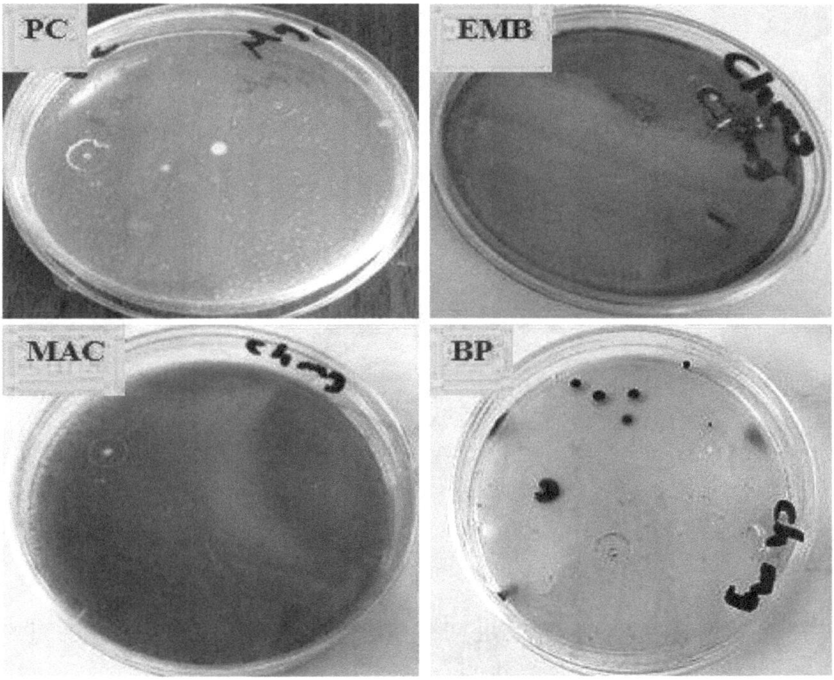

Figure 13: Different bacterial colonies isolated from *Chrysomya megacephala* during the bloated stage [209]

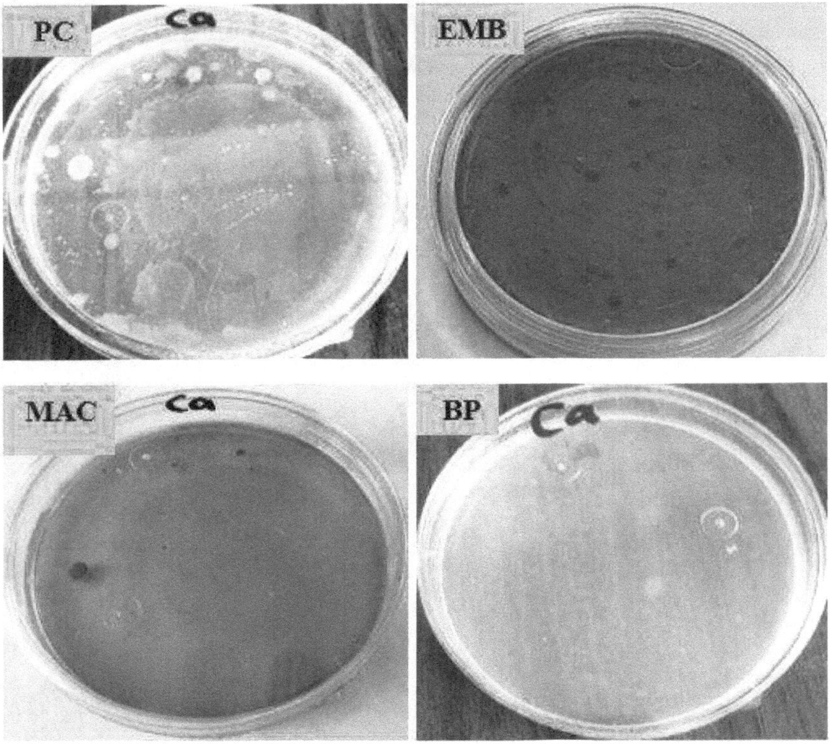

Figure 14: Different bacterial colonies isolated from *Calliphora sp* during the decay stage [209]

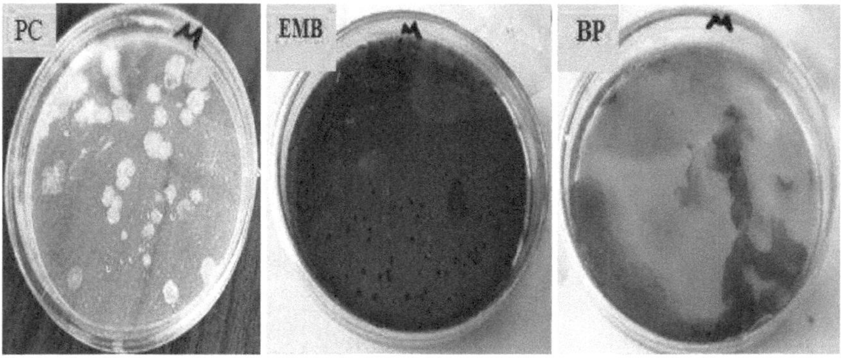

Figure 15: Different bacterial colonies isolated from *Musca domestica* during the fresh stage [209]

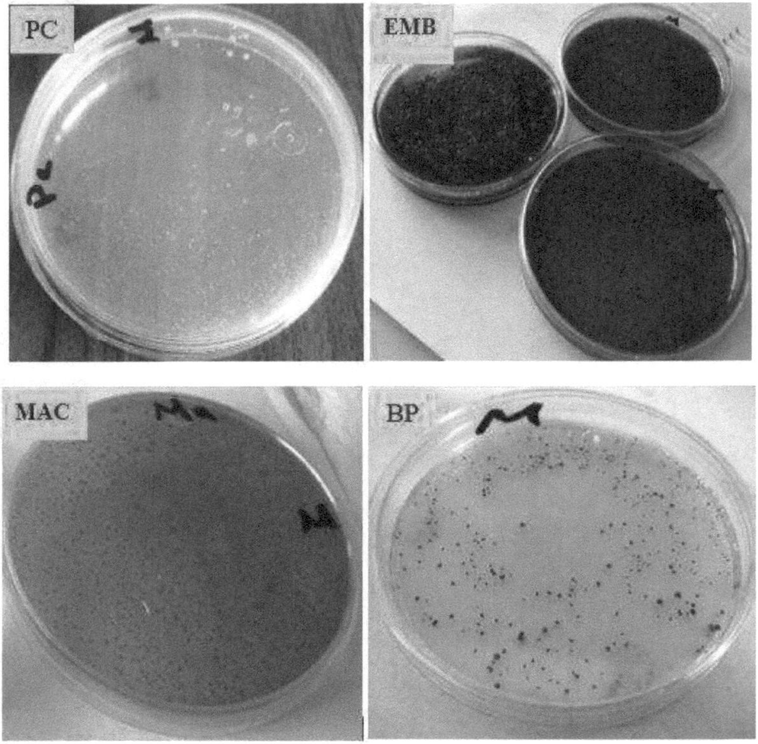

Figure 16: Different bacterial colonies isolated from *Musca domestica* during the bloated stage [209]

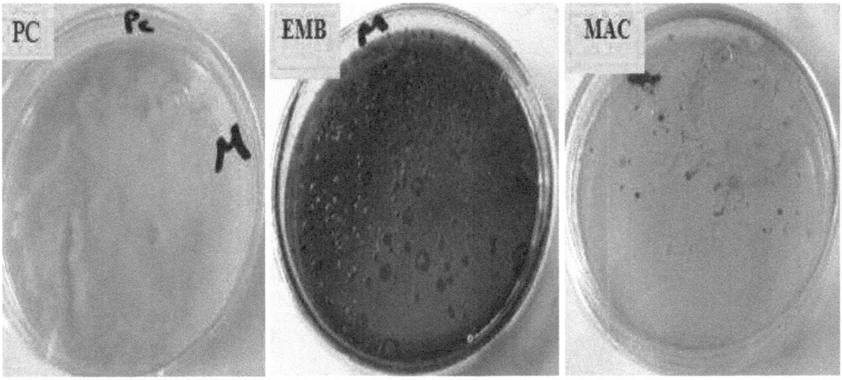

Figure 17: Different bacterial colonies isolated from *Musca domestica* during the decay stage.[209]

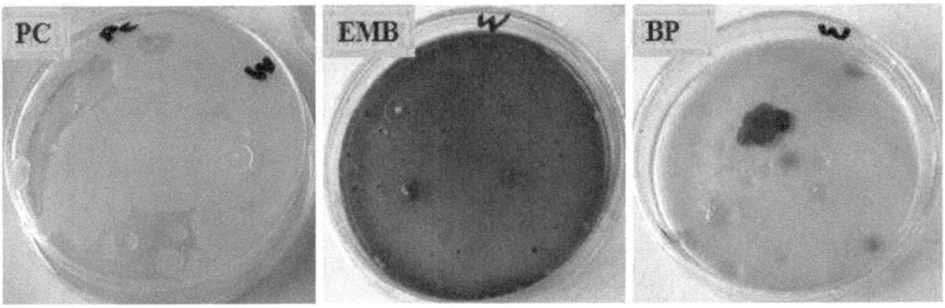

Figure 18: Different bacterial colonies isolated from *Wohlfartia magnifica* during the fresh stage [209]

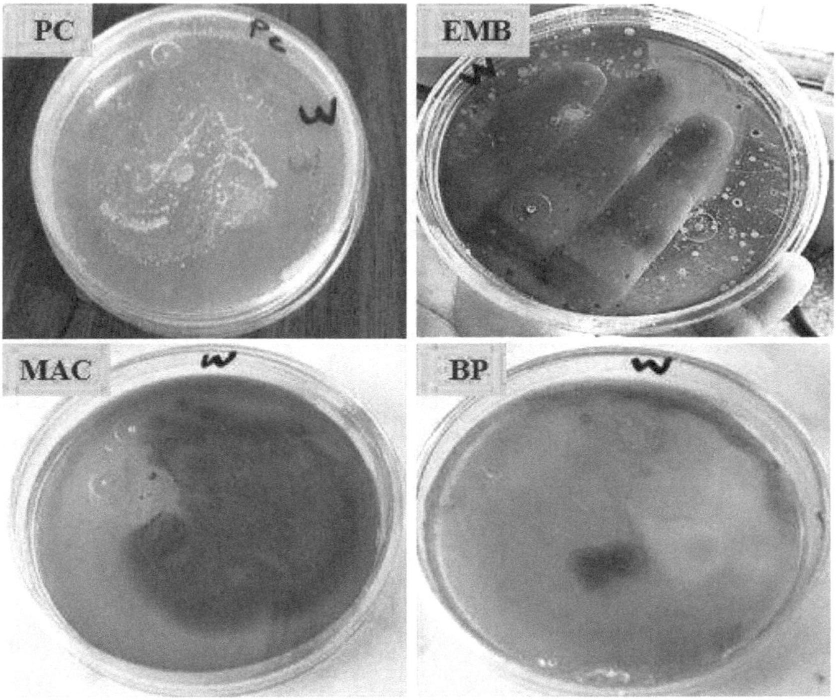

Figure 19: Different bacterial colonies isolated from *Wohlfartia magnifica* during the bloated stage [209]

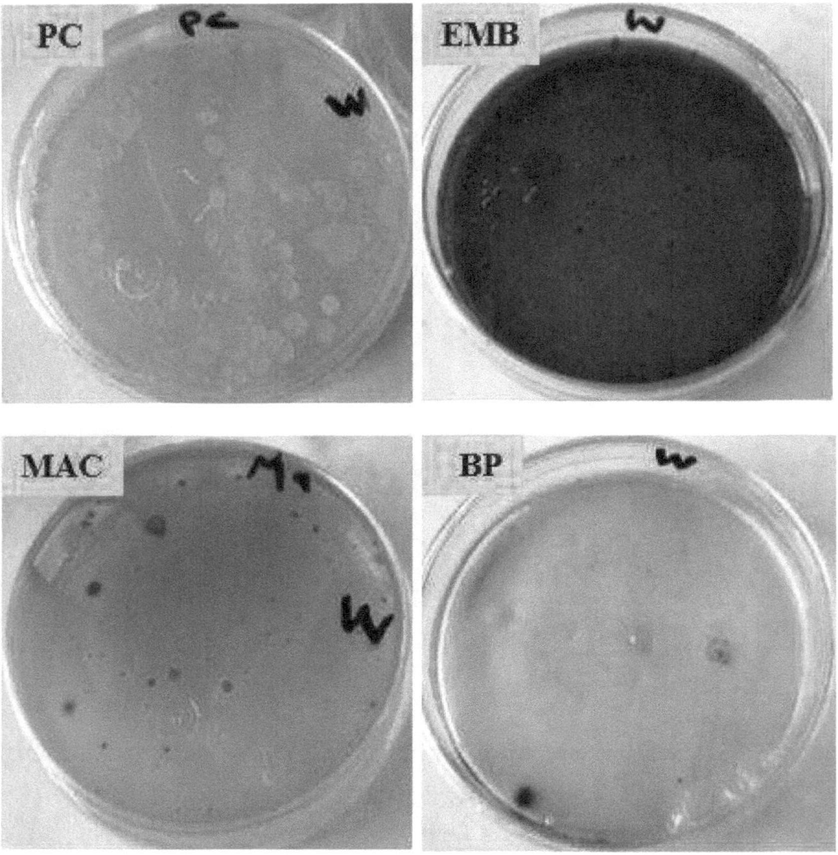

Figure 20: Different bacterial colonies isolated from *Wohlfartia magnifica* during the decay stage [209]

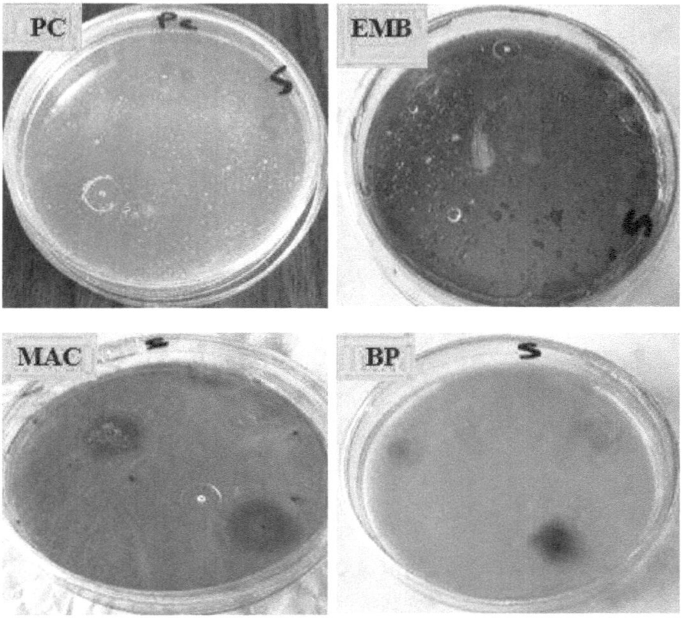

Figure 21: Different bacterial colonies isolated from *Sarcophaga carnaria* during a bloated stage [209]

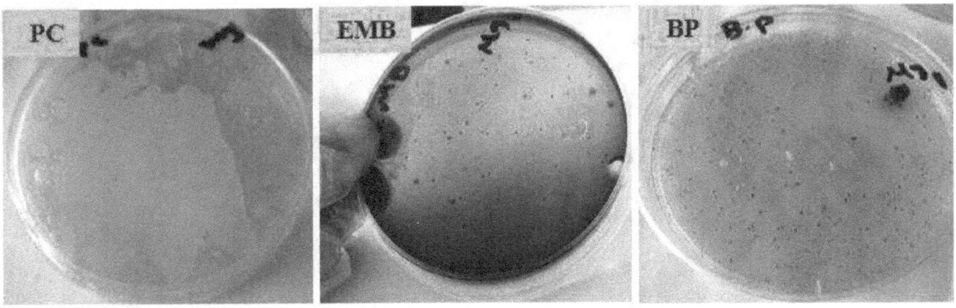

Figure 22: Different bacterial colonies isolated from the external body surface of *Piophila casei* during the decay stage [209]

Many studies serve as a foundational element for examining the bacterial diversity of flies that cause myiasis in connection with rabbit carcasses. Previous research has delved into the use of forensic insects on various animal remains, such as cats, dogs, pigs, guinea pigs, mice, rabbits, and dogs. Additionally, Azwandi *et al.* conducted an assessment of the diversity of arthropod phyla on rat, rabbit, and long-tail monkey carcasses, revealing discrepancies in the species collected. The studies also identified similar variations in the number of species found on rabbit carcasses [207- 217]. The findings of the other research indicated that Calliphoridae were more prevalent in the initial stages of decomposition, while Sarcophagidae dominated in the later stages. These results align with previous studies by De Carvalho and Linhares, who used pig carcasses, and Zeariya *et al.*, who used rabbit and dog carcasses. The study also identified *Musca domestica*, *Chrysomya albiceps*, and *Wohlfartia magnifica* as the most frequently observed flies during the decomposition process of rabbit carcasses [218].

The findings align with prior research conducted by Payne and Zeariya *et al.*, which highlighted the integral role that Blow flies, particularly *Chrysomya albiceps*, play in the decomposition of carcasses. These flies reaffirm their significance as key contributors to carcass decomposition. Turner's study revealed that each stage of decomposition attracts different species due to the various environmental factors present around the carrion. Additionally, Kaiko and Stappenbeck noted that the successful breakdown of animal tissues relies on intricate microbial interactions and successions, which can be influenced by environmental conditions. Insects and microbes consistently partake in ongoing activities throughout this process, leading to active decay. Furthermore, enteric soil bacteria are known to play a crucial role in the decomposition of animal tissues [219- 223].

According to Mohammed *et al.*, the advanced stage of deterioration commences once the majority of muscoid fly larvae have vacated the carcass. The internal organ structure is reduced to a mushy substance. After the consumption and desiccation of this material, the dry residues phase begins. Several factors such as insect activity, population, geographical location, temperature, humidity, rainfall, habitat, season, and size and type of the carcass influence the duration of each stage. Research demonstrating the significant role of flies in the decomposition process effectively measured both the accessibility of carrion to insects and the absence of insects from carrion. The gradual decomposition of the carcass attracted flies, beetles, ants, and a variety of other insects. The succession patterns of carrion-arthropods, which illustrate how the nature and composition of fauna change over the course of decay, represent another analytical approach [224- 226].

Authors used various types of agar medium in this study, such as plate count agar for general purpose enrichment, Eosin methylene blue agar and MacConkey agar for selective and differential culturing of Gram-Negative bacteria, and Baird Parker agar for Gram-positive bacteria. One commonly used method for assessing microbial diversity is selective and differential plating followed by viable counts, which provides information on the culturable portion of the microbial population. Selective media can also be useful for identifying and isolating specific microorganisms with particular characteristics, whether beneficial or pathogenic, in a cost-effective manner. Early studies on microbial communities heavily relied on traditional cultural techniques and primarily focused on pathogenic strains [227- 229]. Several comprehensive evaluations utilizing culture-independent techniques have been conducted recently to study bacterial communities in various insects. Flies are particularly intriguing due to their reproduction in decaying organic matter, which harbors a diverse array of microorganisms. The selection of suitable nutrient sources and the establishment of optimal growth conditions pose limitations on the implementation of these methodologies, including factors such as temperature, pH, and oxygen availability. The flies exhibited significant contamination by various pathogenic bacteria [230- 232].

The bacteria included *Staphylococcus epidermidis*, Staphylococcus hominis, Staphylococcus warneri, *Staphylococcus sciuri*, *Escherichia coli*, *Klebsiella pneumonia*e subspecies pneumonia, *Pseudomonas aeruginosa*, and *Proteus mirabilis* increased risk of diseases that transmission through flies. These results align closely with those of Mohammed *et al.* [233], who conducted an ecological study on zoonotic bacteria spread by flies in cow farms and *found Escherichia coli* (*E. coli*), *Staphylococcus aureus*, *Enterobacter*, Staphylococci, *Klebsiella* sp., *Salmonella* spp., *Shigella* spp., and *Proteus* spp. were the most common bacterial isolates. Fouda *et al.* [232] isolated and identified 11 bacterial strains from *Musca domestica*, *Chrysomya albiceps*, and *Lucilia sericata* adults associated with varying carrion. The presence of *E. coli* and other Enterobacterales raises significant public health concerns as this bacterium has been linked to cases of gastroenteritis. *Staphylococcus* spp., *Bacillus* spp., and *E. coli* are known to produce potent enterotoxins leading to rapid-onset diseases characterized by symptoms such as nausea, vomiting, and diarrhea within a few hours [234]. The findings corroborate prior research that identified Enterobacterales as the predominant species isolated from various insects. Despite their prevalence, Enterobacterales are not the exclusive taxon present on the external surface of collected flies. Furthermore, Förster *et al.* conducted a laboratory experiment on synanthropic flies, including *Musca*, *Sarcophaga*, *Calliphora*, *Fannia*, *Lucilia*, and *Stomoxys*, as potential carriers of virulent microbes. Their study concluded that different fly species were associated with foodborne and other infections. The common house fly, *Musca domestica*, has long been considered a potential vector for epidemics. Butler *et al.* examined the transmission of harmful bacteria by wild Florida house flies (*Musca domestica*). Among the newly discovered bacteria associated with house flies were *Acinetobacter baumanni*, *Bacillus pumilus*, *Cronobacter sakazakii*, *Methylobacterium persicinum*, and *Staphylococcus sciuri*. Others like *Bacillus cereus*, *Bacillus thuringiensis*, *Escherichia coli* 0157:H7, *Shigella dysenteriae*, *Staphylococcus saprophyticus*, and *Staphylococcus xylosus* have also been previously linked to house flies [235-239]. Choo *et al.* further investigated the extraction of *Campylobacter* and *Salmonella* from *Musca domestica*, emphasizing the role of insects such as house flies and cockroaches in disseminating pathogens that contribute to the spread of diseases in both agricultural settings and human populations, specifically *Salmonella* spp. and *Campylobacters* [240]. Moreover, Chaiwong *et al.* conducted a study on the *Chrysomya megacephala* (*Chrysomya megacephala*) and found that the bacteria most commonly isolated from this species were streptococci and staphylococci. It was observed that *C. megacephala* has the potential to transfer harmful intestinal bacteria to humans. In a separate study by Habeeb and Mahdi, the mechanical transmission of bacteria by true fly species was investigated, with the isolation of 18 different bacterial species including *E. coli*, *Staphylococcus*, *Streptococcus*, and *Enterobacter* from various Muscidae, Calliphoridae, and *Sarcophagidae* species in different areas of Lahore City. The research indicated that acute gastroenteritis presents a significant public health concern. *Musca domesticat* has been identified as a host for infectious diseases, acting as a vector for helminths, bacteria, protozoa, viruses, and various parasites that have implications for public health [240- 246].

Identification of bacteria by Vitek 2 system

The Vitek 2 system utilized Analytical Profile Indexes to identify various bacterial species. This system successfully categorized 40 bacterial isolates across 5 different genera, including *Staphylococcus epidermidis*, *Staphylococcus hominis*, *Staphylococcus warneri*, *Staphylococcus sciuri*, *Escherichia coli* (*E. coli*), *Klebsiella pneumonia*e, *Pseudomonas aeruginosa*, and *Proteus mirabilis* [246]. Among these, *E. coli* was the most commonly identified bacterial isolate, making up 40% of the total. The percentage distribution of virulent bacterial species found in forensic flies in relation to different stages of rabbit carcass decomposition was studied. The reliability of the identification profiles was deemed to be high. The Vitek 2 system's methodology for organism identification is based on data analysis and a thorough understanding of the organism's characteristics and analytical reactions. This system has gathered adequate data from known strains to predict how the claimed species typically react to a variety of distinguishing biochemicals [246].

Studying the colonization patterns of insects and microbial communities in buried remains of forensic significance

In numerous instances of violent criminal activity, the perpetrator frequently attempts to hide the crime and eliminate the victim's body through burial, typically creating superficial graves due to the bulk and mass of a human body. Consequently, buried remains are subject to various variables that influence decomposition and ultimately the estimation of the postmortem interval (PMI). These variables may include abiotic conditions such as soil pH, temperature, type, and moisture, as well as biotic factors like environmental microbial populations and access to insect colonizers [247, 248].

When estimating the postmortem interval for buried remains, it is crucial to consider the influence of biotic factors such as microbial and insect dynamics during decomposition. Previous research has primarily focused on the insect and bacterial species involved in decomposition using surface remains. Therefore, the present study sought to examine the decomposition of buried rat carcasses as a model for human cadavers [249- 257].

Various research studies have been conducted in several countries including Great Britain, Poland, Australia, Argentina, the United States, Canada, Germany, and South Africa to investigate the decomposition process of buried remains. Many of these studies utilized human cadavers and pig carcasses, with a few using juvenile rat and sheep carcasses for experimental purposes; however, there was a lack of comprehensive analysis of the bacterial and insect communities involved. These studies explored various aspects of decomposition, ranging from initial observations of decay in different soil types to patterns of colonization by necrophagous insect species, and most recently, the characterization of the necrobiome structure for potential forensic applications [258-278].

The process of carcass decomposition in the soil varies from decomposition that occurs on the surface. The surface remains typically show clear stages of decomposition such as fresh, bloat, active decay, advanced decay, and finally skeletal remains. Similarly, buried remains can also undergo distinct stages of decomposition starting with the fresh stage, where the abdomen begins to swell, followed by primary and secondary bloat stages characterized by gas buildup and unpleasant odours. Subsequently, as the abdomen deflates, the remains progress to the active decay stage where tissues are still intact, with decomposers and scavengers actively breaking down the remains [279, 280].

As the remains decompose and desiccate, the presence of liquids diminishes or disappears, potentially leading to the formation of adipocere as the remains undergo the transformation into skeletal remains. Additionally, the decomposition process of both surface and buried remains is significantly influenced by various taphonomic factors, including pre-mortem circumstances such as covering or clothing, injuries, environmental elements like the type of burial site and soil composition, time of year, temperature variations, and the presence of insects and scavengers [281].

Temperature fluctuation is a key factor that impacts the decomposition of carcasses, with an optimal range of 20–40 °C for tissue breakdown, particularly at 36°C. Extreme temperatures below 10°C or above 40°C can hinder the decomposition process. Climate variations also influence insect activity and the likelihood of carcass colonization in soil. The decomposition of buried carcasses is influenced by oxygen levels, with low levels affecting microbial community composition and slowing down the process by impacting insect colonization. When studying buried locations, environmental variables such as depth, geographical location, season, and meteorological conditions must be taken into account, along with soil composition and chemistry as crucial factors for decomposition [282, 283].

Moreover, the composition of soil necrophagous entomofauna differs significantly from that found on surface remains, with varying dominant families in terms of both quantity and diversity. Unlike the predominant Calliphoridae family found on surface remains, buried carcasses tend to attract a higher number of specimens belonging to the Phoridae and Muscidae families. The process of colonization occurs when necrophagous insects lay their eggs on the surface of the soil or navigate through the soil to reach the carcass. This behaviour can be influenced by factors such as season, temperature, soil texture, and burial depth. Previous studies have indicated that Phoridae, Muscidae, and Sarcophagidae are the most common species recovered from buried remains [283- 285].

Case reports describing necrophagous insects found on buried bodies are limited, as most studies focus on exhumed remains. In addition, the emerging field of forensic microbiology aims to address challenges in estimating postmortem intervals by studying changes in the microbial community structure. These investigations examine the necrobiome structure of vertebrate carcasses, microbial community shifts during decomposition, and the soil microbial and fungal communities associated with the body. Overall, forensic microbiology aims to enhance postmortem interval estimation alongside forensic entomology by applying similar principles [286-293]. However, research on the microbiome of decomposing organisms and insect microbiomes has predominantly concentrated on surface remains, with fewer studies examining buried remains. While these studies have been instrumental in understanding the decomposition process, they have primarily been conducted in laboratory settings or have solely explored the variety of bacterial communities associated with soil [294- 296].

The studies indicate that the microbial communities in soil, associated with hosts, and associated with insects undergo changes as decomposition progresses. The focus of forensic investigations is on the ability to monitor these changes over time, leading to research efforts to understand both the general shifts in the community over time and the specific changes in certain members of these communities that could serve as indicators of postmortem interval. For example, a study examining particular taxa within the human gut microbiome observed that certain taxa could be traced throughout the process of decomposition [296].

Specifically, *Bacteroides* sp., *Lactobacillus* sp., and *Bifidobacterium* sp. were measured using qPCR during the decomposition of human bodies as potential quantitative markers of PMI. Additional research on quantitative analysis of the Firmicutes phylum has focused on examining water samples or the overall gut microbiota [297- 299].

In order to gain a deeper comprehension of the contributions of insects and microbes in the decomposition of buried remains and their implications for postmortem interval estimation, this study offers a thorough examination of both insects and bacteria as key decomposers, as well as the environmental variables that may impact the process. Rat carcasses were utilized as substitutes for human remains to monitor shifts in insect populations and microbial communities. The use of rat carcasses as analogues benefits from their widespread usage in clinical human studies, allowing for greater replication and easier collection of samples compared to human tissue [297].

Previous forensic experiments have demonstrated the suitability of rodents as models due to the similarity in decomposition processes and microbial compositions between rat carcasses and human cadavers. The research was conducted over two 30-day periods in spring and summer (March and June) in a temperate continental climate region in Eastern Europe (Bucharest, Romania). The primary goals of the study were to qualitatively and quantitatively assess the necrophagous insect population and the necrobiome during the decomposition process using buried rat carcasses, as well as to analyze the environmental factors influencing decomposition and describe the colonization patterns of key decomposers. A comprehensive understanding of the colonization behaviour of necrophagous insect species and the bacterial communities associated with carcasses and insects is crucial for determining accurate postmortem interval estimations for buried remains [300- 305].

The specimens were humanely euthanized through carbon dioxide inhalation as per both international and national regulations, including EU Directive 86–609-EEC 2010/63/EU and law number 43/2014, and were approved by the ethical committee of the Institute of Biology Bucharest, the location of the analyses. The carcasses were interred in shallow graves at a depth of 40 cm, spaced at least 0.5 m apart, and left exposed to the natural environment without any coverings or barriers. Rat carcasses were selected as human substitutes due to their ability to provide a greater number of specimens for replication and being a widely accepted animal model for human biological studies. Furthermore, previous research has shown rat carcasses to be effective experimental models in decomposition studies [306- 308].

Temperature, humidity, and soil conditions were monitored at regular intervals using sophisticated thermo-hygrometers, while precipitation data was sourced from the National Meteorological Administration. The pH levels of the soil were measured daily utilizing advanced equipment. Control sites were established to monitor pH levels and insect activity in the absence of rat carcasses at a specific depth. Exposed carcasses were not utilized as burial controls as the focus of the study was on documenting the organisms present on buried remains and analyzing the impact on gut communities [309]. Each rat carcass was excavated meticulously using a short-handled wooden spade. The specimens were sampled destructively in triplicate by extracting a portion of the small intestine, which was then preserved in 200 µl Tris-EDTA pH 8 (TE) buffer at −20 °C before discarding the carcass. A total of thirty rat carcasses were utilized for each month. Necrophagous insect species, including both adults and larvae, were daily observed and collected in June using an entomological net and forceps. The specimens were stored in 200 µl Tris-EDTA pH 8 (TE) buffer at −20 °C for DNA extraction, while taxonomic identification was conducted using 75% ethanol. Larvae were placed in rearing jars during each sampling period, although none survived to pupate. Pupae found on the rat carcasses were collected and kept under constant temperature and humidity until they hatched. Due to the low temperatures in March, no insects were able to be collected. Taxonomic and genetic identification of necrophagous insect species was carried out. Adult and immature insects were taxonomically identified using a Stereomicroscope Leica S6D (Leica Microsystems, Wetzlar, Germany) along with identification keys provided by Disney64, Gregor *et al.*, and Grzywacz *et al.* DNA barcoding was conducted by amplifying the COI (Cytochrome C Oxidase I) gene fragment from the insects [310-312]. Before proceeding with DNA extraction, an additional step involving cell disruption using 2 mm ZR Bashing Beads from Zymo Research in Irvine, CA, USA, was conducted with a SpeedMill PLUS Cell Homogenizer from Analitik Jena in Jena, Germany, set at 20 °C and 50 Hz-power for a duration of 12 minutes. The total DNA was then extracted following the manufacturer's protocol from the DNeasy Blood & Tissue Kit provided by Qiagen in Valencia, CA, USA. Subsequent to extraction, the DNA purity and concentration were assessed using a

Biodrop spectrophotometer from Denville Scientific Inc in Holliston, MA, USA, and amplified using a Mastercycler ProS System from Eppendorf in Wien, Austria. The PCR process was carried out in a total volume of 50 µl, incorporating 200 ng/µl of insect DNA, 10 pmol/ml each of the forward LCO1490 and reverse HC02198 primers, 0.1 mM dNTP, 1U of Taq DNA polymerase, and 1x Taq buffer with 2.5 mM $MgCl_2$ from ThermoFisher Scientific in Waltham, MA, USA. The DNA amplification comprised various steps including denaturation, annealing, and extension at specified temperatures for specific durations. The resulting DNA fragments of 710 bp were scrutinized on 1% agarose gels from Cleaver Scientific in Rugby, UK, alongside a negative control. The Polymerase chain reaction (PCR) products were then purified using the PureLink PCR Purification Kit from ThermoFisher Scientific before being sent for sequencing to Macrogen Genomics in the Netherlands. The validation of insect COI nucleotide sequences coverage and identity was conducted utilizing BLAST-NCBI69. The sequences were then subjected to quality trimming and alignment using Sequence Assembly and Alignment Software - CodonCode. The identified sequences were deposited in the GenBank database under the accession numbers: [KY582492, KY582507, KY582509] for *Muscina prolapsa* third instar larvae, adult, and teneral specimen (Diptera: Muscidae); [KY582497] for *Muscina levida* third instar larvae (Diptera: Muscidae); [KY582504] for *Hydrotaea ignava* third instar larvae (Diptera: Muscidae), listed in GenBank as leucostoma; [KY582493, KY582496] for *Megaselia rufipes* (Diptera: Phoridae) larvae and adult; [KY582506] for *Leiodidae* sp. (*Coleoptera*) adult; and [KY582503] for *Medon brunneus* (Coleoptera: Staphylinidae) [313-316].

16S rRNA gene sequencing was conducted using the Illumina platform to analyze bacterial communities. The DNA was extracted from rat tissue and insects as per established protocol and the concentration was determined with a Qubit fluorometer. PCR amplification of 16S rRNA gene fragments from the V3-V4 variable region was carried out with primer pair 341F/806R71 from McGill University and Génome Québec Innovation Centre. The barcoded amplicons were analyzed in triplicate, combined in equal amounts, and sequenced on the Illumina MiSeq PE300 platform at the same centre. The sequences were quality-filtered at a q-score of 30 and merged in PEAR (v0.9.5) with a cut-off length of 300 base pairs [317, 318]. The remaining sequences were deduplicated, and individual sequences that appeared only once were eliminated using USEARCH73 through Quantitative Insights into Microbial Ecology (QIIME). The sequences were grouped into operational taxonomic units (OTUs) using UPARSE73. Each OTU was represented by the most prevalent sequence in the cluster, which served as the reference database for aligning the original sequences with a 97% similarity threshold and assigning taxonomy based on the QIIME-formatted SILVA database. The number of sequences per sample ranged from 188 to 235,295, with a mean and median of 137,471 and 141,646 sequences, respectively. One set of triplicates from one sample (IP 14.2) was excluded from the final dataset due to its low sequencing depth of 188 sequences and lack of taxonomy assignment. Ultimately, the final dataset included a total of 2,049 OTUs from 69 samples. This data represents the complete dataset for this decomposition experiment. A subset of this data was used to describe a previously unobserved necrophagous insect in Romania [319-321].

Quantitative polymerase chain reaction (qPCR)

The standard method for detecting nucleic acids in all fields of microbiology, biomedical research, biotechnology, and forensic applications is the real-time fluorescence-based quantitative polymerase chain reaction (qPCR). The quantitative polymerase chain reaction (qPCR) was used to determine many bacteria like *Enterococcus faecalis* (*E. faecalis*) and *Clostridium paraputrificum* (*C. paraputrificum*) which abundances during decomposition was conducted through qPCR using specific primers: ENTFRev/ENTFFw51 for *E. faecalis* and CLPARev/CLPAFw77 for *C. paraputrificum*. A 10 µl reaction volume containing Thermo Scientific Maxima SYBR Green qPCR Master Mix (2x), 0.3 µM of each forward and reverse primer, 200 ng template DNA, and nuclease-free water was utilized for the amplification reactions. The reactions were performed in a Mastercycler ep gradient S thermocycler PCR, with an initial incubation at 95 °C for 10 min followed by 40 cycles of amplification (15 sec at 95 °C, 30 sec at 55 °C for *E. faecalis* or 56 °C for *C. paraputrificum*, and 30 sec at 72 °C). After each program, a melting curve analysis was conducted to confirm the production of the desired amplicon by the SYBR green assay. Quantification was achieved by interpolation on a standard regression curve of cycle threshold (Ct) values obtained from DNA templates of known concentrations. The PCR product from a previous reaction, purified from a 1% agarose gel and quantified using a BiodropDuo UV/VIS Spectrophotometer, was used as the template for the standard curve. Decimal dilutions of DNA concentrations ranging from 3.7–3.7 × 10−4 ng/uL for *E. faecalis* and 3.9–3.9 × 10−4 ng/uL for *C. paraputrificum* were prepared for the standard curve. Standard curves were constructed by plotting Ct values versus log10 (ng DNA/reaction), with a requirement of R2 > 0.99 for consideration. Real-time PCR assays with Cycle Threshold (Ct) values exceeding

40 were categorized as negative. To ensure accuracy, non-template controls were included in all PCR runs and yielded negative results. Each sample was meticulously analyzed in triplicate, with two rounds of amplification performed for each individual sample. The quantification of genome copies of DNA was determined using established formulas as outlined by Clifford and colleagues. Genome sizes of 3.2 × 106 base pairs (bp) for *E. faecalis* (NCBI_Ref_Seq NC_004668.1) and 3.5 × 106 bp for *C. paraputrificum* (NCBI_Ref_Seq NZ_AUJC01000001.1) were utilized in the calculations. The data was presented as the logarithm (base 10) of the number of genomes per reaction relative to the postmortem days. Statistical analysis was conducted using Microsoft Excel. [322- 324]

The environmental conditions and decomposition process

Environmental conditions were monitored by recording air, soil temperature, and relative humidity using three-button loggers, with soil pH measured in triplicate. Averages with standard error values were then calculated in many studies. The researchers found that in March, the maximum soil and air temperatures reached 10.7 °C and 16.3 °C, respectively, while the minimum thresholds were 7.28 °C and 3.96 °C. The difference between air and soil temperatures varied from 0.04 °C up to 5 °C on the final experimental day. Moving to June, the soil temperature ranged from 16.75 °C to 25.37 °C, with air temperature fluctuating between 15.8 °C and 28.13°C. The discrepancies between the two records were significantly less pronounced, falling within the range of 0.21–2.89 °C [324]. In March, the air relative humidity levels ranged from 52.36% to 99.63%, coinciding with rainfall, while in June, they spanned from 57.13% to 92.2%. March experienced a higher level of precipitation at 10.91 mm, compared to June at 5.08 mm. The soil pH in March ranged from 6.0 to 7.6 for both surrounding soils and grave soil, with the latter seeing an increase to above 8.0 on day 26 while the former remained stable between 6.8 to 7.4. The pH increases in the grave soil corresponded with active and advanced decay stages, although the distinction between them was not clearly defined. In June, pH changes over time were similar for both types of soil, with the grave soil being slightly more alkaline. June witnessed more significant pH fluctuations, with the soil being more acidic during the bloat stage before stabilizing at 6.7 for grave soil and 6.4 for surrounding soil [324]. A significant rise in pH levels was noted in both the soil surrounding the burial site and in the grave soil, correlating with the stages of active decay on day 14 and advanced decay on days 18-21. The process of decomposition displayed notable variations between the two periods under investigation, as illustrated in Figure 23 and 24. In March, characterized by low temperatures and high levels of precipitation, the distinct stages of decomposition were not readily discernible. The initial stage spanned from days 1 to 3, followed by a partial swelling of the abdomen with no apparent discolouration from days 4 to 9 [324].

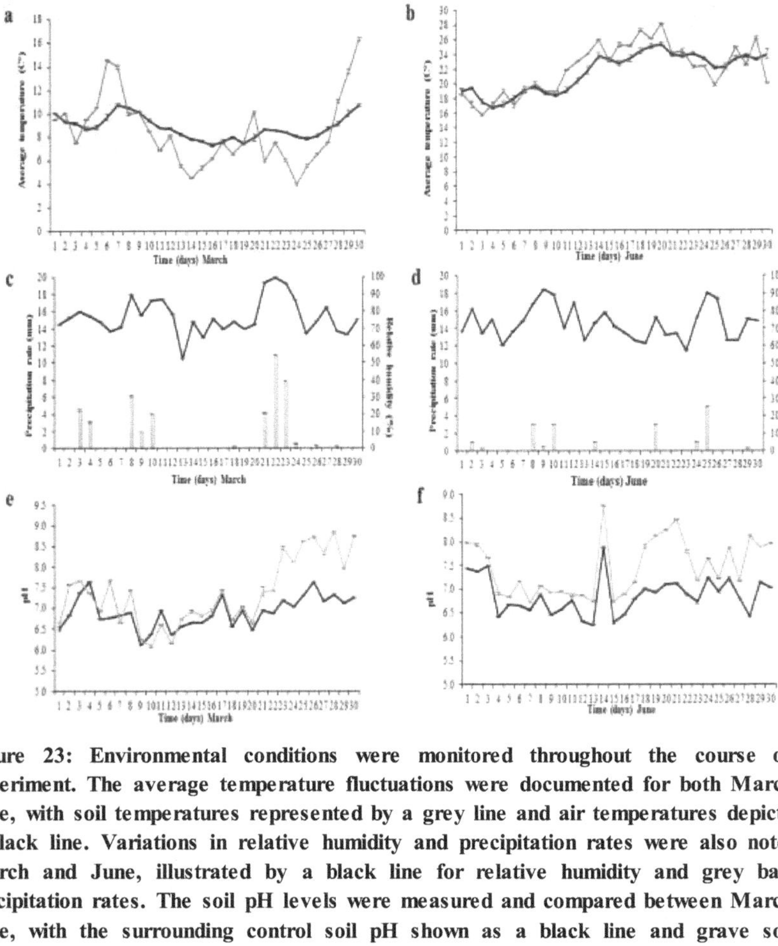

Figure 23: Environmental conditions were monitored throughout the course of the experiment. The average temperature fluctuations were documented for both March and June, with soil temperatures represented by a grey line and air temperatures depicted by a black line. Variations in relative humidity and precipitation rates were also noted for March and June, illustrated by a black line for relative humidity and grey bars for precipitation rates. The soil pH levels were measured and compared between March and June, with the surrounding control soil pH shown as a black line and grave soil pH indicated by a grey line. Standard deviations were calculated and represented by error bars, with a sample size of n=3 [324].

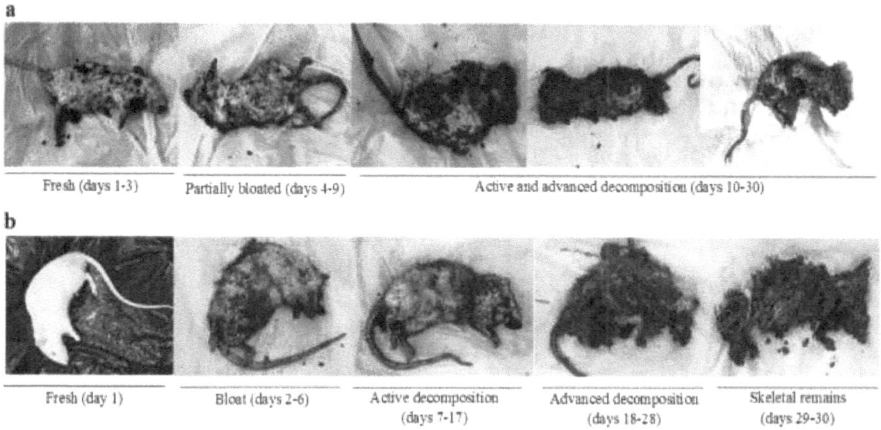

Figure 24: The process of decomposition in buried rat carcasses was observed at different stages, specifically during March and June. On day 10, there was a noticeable separation of the epidermis and fur. By day 18, complete detachment of the fur had occurred, along with a strong odour emanating from the abdominal cavity upon opening. The organs within the abdominal cavity began to display a brownish color and could still be identified until day 25. The small intestine remained intact until day 30, which marked the conclusion of the March experimental period [324].

According to Wilson and colleagues, the decomposition process observed in June can be subdivided into distinct stages. The initial stage was evident on the first day, followed by abdominal bloating, while the build-up of gases became apparent between days 2 and 6. Subsequently, the active decay phase (days 7-17) was characterized by the collapse of the abdominal cavity, a pronounced odor, and the persistence of skin and flesh. From day 18 onwards, the advanced decay stage was indicated by the presence of larvae across the entire carcass surface, with most surface tissues exhibiting high moisture levels until day 25. By days 25 to 30, the majority of organs had liquefied, and the cecum had decomposed, though fragments of the small intestine remained retrievable until day 30 [325]. A Principal Component Analysis (PCA) was employed to investigate the influence of soil temperature, relative humidity, and precipitation rate on the decomposition process in March and June. The PCA utilized the different stages of decomposition as a categorical variable, while soil temperature, relative humidity, and precipitation rate were considered as independent factors. In March, the PCA elucidated 99.9% of the variability across the first two axes (PC1 and PC2), with the third axis explaining less than 1% of the total variance. The first principal component axis exhibited a strong positive correlation with soil temperature, whereas the second principal component axis showed a high association with relative humidity. Similar results were obtained in June, where 99.9% of the variance was captured by the first two axes (PC1 and PC2), and the third axis contributed minimally to the overall variance [325].

Diptera and *Coleoptera* succession

In March, there was no presence of insects due to the cold temperatures. Diptera adults were observed during the active decay stage in June. These specimens were found on the soil surface nine days after burial, although no egg clusters were seen. Three species from the Muscidae family were identified as *Muscina prolapsa*, *Muscina levida*, and *Hydrotaea ignava*. Only third instar larvae of these species were collected for identification. Diptera pupae were observed and collected starting from day 19, with *M. prolapsa* being the only species to emerge from the pupae. Adult emergence typically occurred 7 to 10 days after pupation. An immature *M. prolapsa* specimen was found on day 29. Additionally, two other *Muscidae* species, *M. levida* and *H. ignava*, were observed during different stages of decay [326].

Two species from the Phoridae family, *Megaselia rufipes* and *Conicera similis*, were observed in both larval and adult stages. The presence of *C. similis* is the first documented occurrence in Romania, marking the easternmost location for this species. *C. similis* adults were observed on day 9 and then again on day 25. *Coleoptera* adults from the Staphylinidae and Leiodidae families were observed towards the end of the advanced decay stage on day 26. The *Staphylinidae* species was identified as *Medon brunneus*, while the Leiodidae specimen was only classified at the family level. DNA barcoding confirmed the taxonomic identification of both *Diptera* and *Coleoptera* specimens. For Muscidae, COI amplicons from various life stages showed 100% identity with reference sequences in GenBank. Similarly, Phoridae COI amplicons had 90% identity with reference sequences in GenBank. *Coleoptera* adults from Staphylinidae and Leiodidae also had COI amplicons with high identity to reference sequences (figure 25) [326].

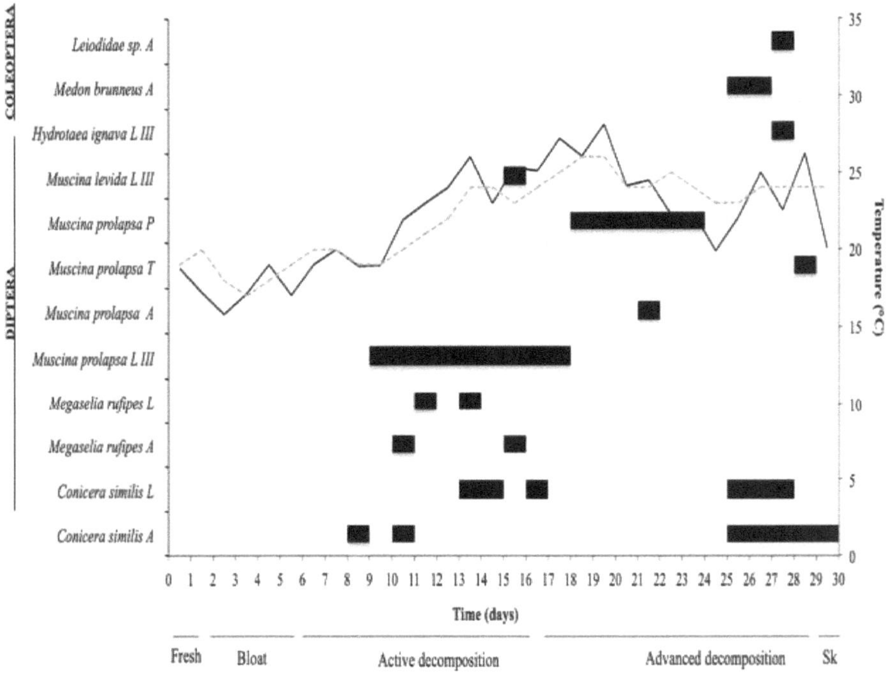

Figure 25: During the June experimental period, the colonization patterns of Diptera (black) and *Coleoptera* (grey) on rat carcasses were observed. Temperature variations in the surrounding soil (grey dashed line) and air (black line), as well as the decomposition stages, were monitored for this specific time frame. Various developmental stages of insects were identified, including adults (A), larvae (L), third instar larvae (LIII), pupae (P), and teneral specimens (T).[326]

16S rRNA Illumina MiSeq characterization of insect and rat small intestine tissues

Analysis of the microbial community profile of necrophagous insect species revealed interesting findings. The bacterial communities linked with third instar *M. prolapsa* were examined during days 12 and 14, corresponding to the active decay stage, day 17 marking the transition between active and advanced decay, and day 26 denoting the end of the advanced decay stage. Furthermore, the bacterial community associated with adult *M. prolapsa* sampled on day 22 and teneral specimens collected on day 29 were also studied [327].

In terms of larval specimens, there was a noticeable increase in Firmicutes during the decomposition process, rising from 13.13% to 41.57%. This corresponded with a decrease in Proteobacteria, especially evident on day 26. The prevalent orders across all insect specimens analyzed were Xanthomonadales, Pseudomonadales, and Clostridiales, with Enterobacteriales, Bacillales, and Corynebacteriales present in lower quantities [327]. The primary families within the Firmicutes and *Proteobacteria* phyla for *M. prolapsa* were identified as Clostridiaceae and Xanthomonadaceae, respectively. Notably, the relative abundance of *Firmicutes* varied significantly between teneral and adult *M. prolapsa* specimens, increasing from 7.00% to 24.97% in adults. Conversely, the relative abundance of *Proteobacteria* increased from larval stages to 54.53% in teneral specimens and 46.60% in adults. *Bacteroidetes*, specifically families Flavobacteriaceae and Sphingobacteriaeae, remained relatively consistent in larval samples until a spike on day 26. *Actinobacter*, particularly families Corynebacteriaceae and Microbacteriaceae, showed an increase in larval samples between days 12-17, followed by a decline on day 26. The teneral specimen exhibited the highest abundance of *Actinobacter*, while the adult had lower levels in comparison. The adult *Coleoptera* specimens, identified as *M. brunneus*, were collected on day 25 (refer to Figure 26). In general, the microbial community of *M. brunneus* closely resembled that of *M. prolapsa*. These microbial communities in adult specimens were mainly comprised of *Proteobacteria* (54.20 (±2.25) %), Firmicutes (18.13 (±1.00) %), and *Actinobacter* (10.63 (±3.78) %). Nevertheless, adult *M. brunneus* exhibited higher levels of *Bacteroidetes* compared to *M. prolapsa* (9.73 (±0.74) %). Both larval and adult samples of *C. similis* were obtained on days 14 and 28, respectively (see Figure 26). Similar to the *M. prolapsa* samples, the larval communities (on day 14) mainly consisted of *Proteobacteria* (50.75 (±0.35) %), *Firmicutes* (22.10 (±3.25)%), and *Actinobacter* (9.50 (±3.11) %). Nevertheless, the larval specimens of *C. similis* showed a higher abundance of *Bacteroidetes* (12.35 (±3.61) %) compared to *M. prolapsa* larvae (4.43 (±0.40) %) [327].

The microbial community composition of the rat small intestine was analyzed. The initial samples collected in March exhibited microbial communities with a high, yet variable, proportion of *Proteobacteria* (70.87 (±44.83) %) and a low, yet variable, proportion of Firmicutes (6.93 (±10.89) %) (refer to Supplementary Figure S1). Following day 2, there was a noticeable shift in phyla where Firmicutes increased while *Proteobacteria* decreased (88.57 (±3.59%) and 3.60 (±2.07) %, respectively). Subsequently, from days 5 to 10, there was a decrease in Firmicutes and an increase in *Proteobacteria*, which once again changed on day 18. As the decomposition progressed towards its advanced stage, on day 25, *Proteobacteria* became the dominant phylum (71.61 (±10.04) %) but was then overtaken by Firmicutes on the final day of the experiment as the primary phylum (33.10 (±1.95) %). Additionally, *Actinobacteria*, *Bacteroidetes*, and *Acidobacteria* were also present in the microbial community [327].

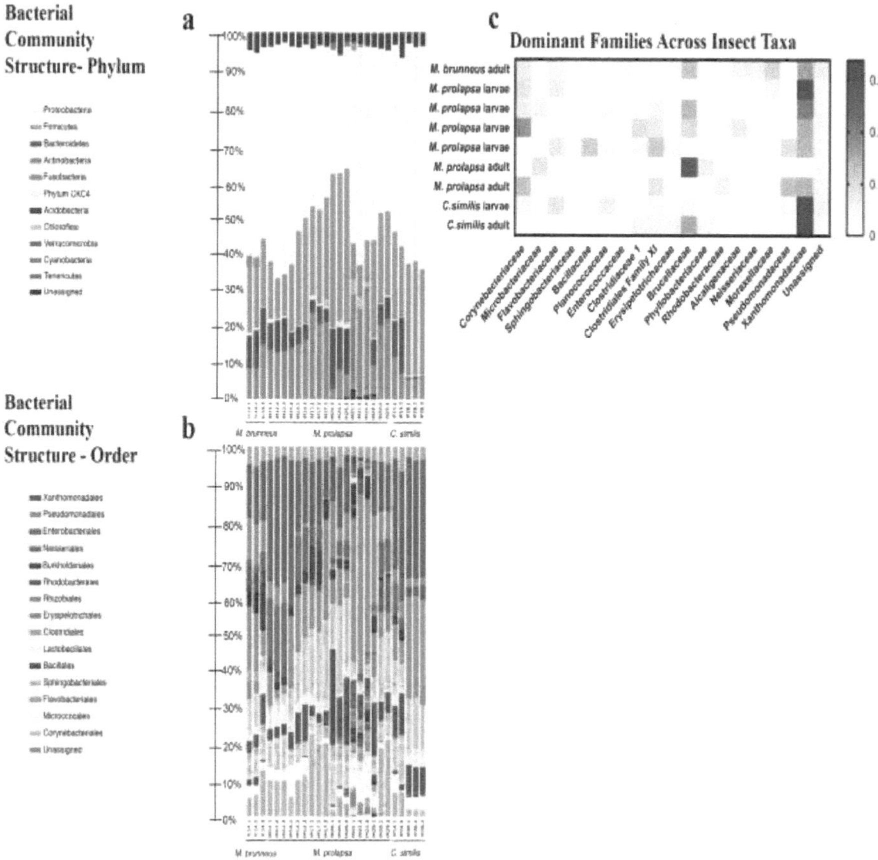

Figure 26. The bacterial diversity of samples associated with insects was analyzed based on phylum, order, and family. Within the phylum level, various orders were identified in the samples. The orders were further classified into families, including Staphylinidae, Muscidae, and Phoridae. The specific species identified within each family were *M. brunneus* for Staphylinidae, *M. prolapsa* for Muscidae, and *C. similis* for Phoridae [327].

In March, alterations in the relative abundance of bacterial communities can be defined by the trade-off between phyla *Firmicutes* and *Proteobacteria* during decomposition, alongside the consistent but low levels of *Actinobacter*, *Bacteroidetes*, and *Acidobacteria*. Conversely, in early June, Firmicutes dominated the community composition at 97.77%, unlike the situation in March. Within the early stages of decomposition in June, there was a notable presence of *Actinobacter* at 24.23% despite some variability. Throughout the active decomposition stages on days 7 and 12, Firmicutes and Proteobacteria levels remained similar to March samples, while Fusobacteria increased significantly during advanced decay, reaching a peak relative abundance of 39.90%. Overall, the bacterial community composition in June was characterized by the prevalence of Firmicutes, with other phyla diminishing over time or exhibiting brief increases followed by dissipation. At the order level, Clostridiales and Lactobacillales were more prominent in early decomposition stages in both March and June, while Enterobacteriales were observed later in the decay process. Fusobacteriales increased during advanced decay, with Bacteroidiales showing an increase towards the end of decomposition. Major families within the experimental period included Helicobacteraceae, Enterobacteriaceae, and Peptostreptococcacae. Evaluating the overall diversity of microbial communities in insect and rat intestines, it was found that insect larval samples exhibited higher richness in alpha diversity compared to adult samples. Furthermore, insect communities showed greater richness and diversity in alpha diversity compared to rat intestines. Variations were observed not only within samples but also between them, indicating different bacterial communities. The total diversity of taxa remained consistent between the two experimental periods, with March showing 23 phyla, 103 orders, and 410 genera, and June exhibiting 23 phyla, 95 orders, and 374 genera. Pearson's correlation analysis conducted to explore the variation among microbial communities in relation to pH and Shannon diversity revealed no significant correlation between bacterial diversity and pH ($p = 0.41$, $r2 = 0.06$) (Figure 27) [328].

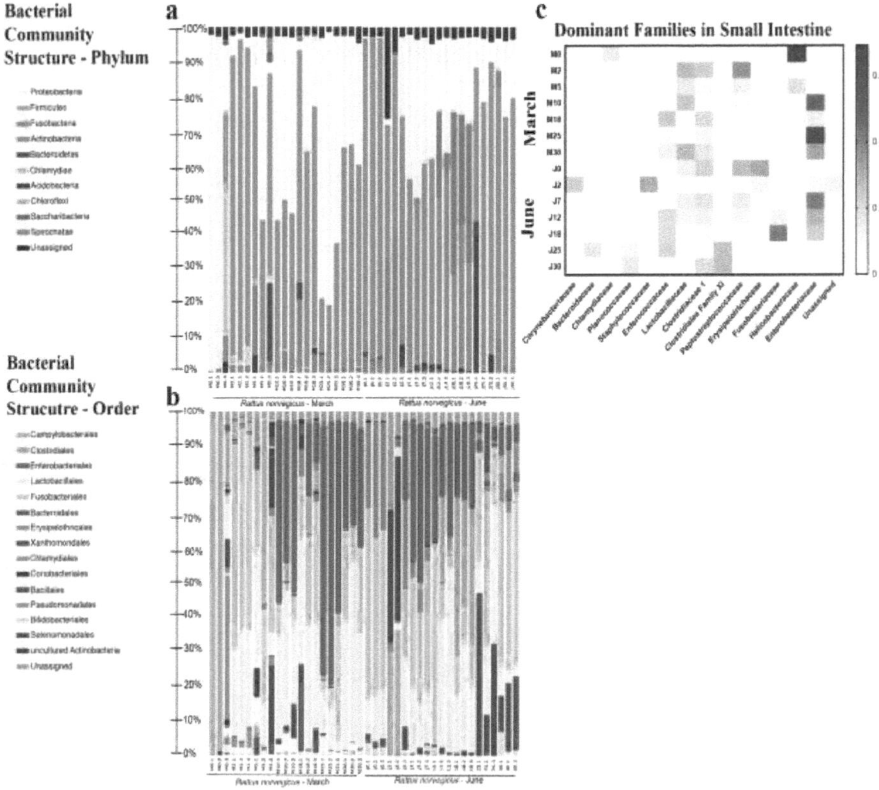

Figure 27: The composition of bacterial communities in samples associated with the intestines of rats was analyzed, with a focus on phylum, order, and family level taxa that were present in at least 1.0% of the total dataset across different time points [328].

Enterococcus faecalis and *Clostridium paraputrificum* postmortem relative abundances

Due to the prevalence of phylum Firmicutes in the human gut microbiome and their frequent presence during human decomposition, *Enterococcus faecalis* and *Clostridium paraputrificum* were chosen for quantitative analysis in order to identify potential postmortem microbial markers for estimating time since death (Figure 28). For *Enterococcus faecalis*, the abundance varied across the experiments conducted in March and June, with the highest bacterial content observed at different stages of decomposition, reaching 102.5 during advanced decay and 104.5 during active decay. In March, a logarithmic increase in bacterial levels was noted from the fresh stage to the initial active decomposition phase (days 1–13), which then stabilized for the remainder of the experimental period (days 13–30). Conversely, in June, a swift rise in *E. faecalis* abundance occurred during the fresh and bloat stages (days 1–6), leveling off during the early active decomposition phase (days 7–30) with minimal fluctuations. While the initial amount of *E. faecalis* in the rat intestines during the March experiment was approximately five times lower than in June, the changes in abundance of this species towards the latter stages of carcass decay were consistent (103.5 ± 102.19). However, the growth of *E. faecalis* during the initial stages of decomposition seemed to be heavily influenced by environmental factors, particularly soil temperature. *Clostridium paraputrificum* was first detected during March on day 8 postmortem, corresponding to the active and advanced decomposition phases. The relative abundance of this species (101.1) was significantly lower compared to that of *E. faecalis* (103.4) and displayed an overall decline throughout the decomposition process [327].

In June, the occurrence of this particular species was limited, making it difficult to determine a definitive pattern. This species was only observed during the period of active decay, typically occurring between days 11 and 15 after death. The process of decomposition in buried remains, whether they be a human or non-human mammal, has not received as much research attention as the surface remains, particularly in relation to necrophagous insects and the necrobiome [327].

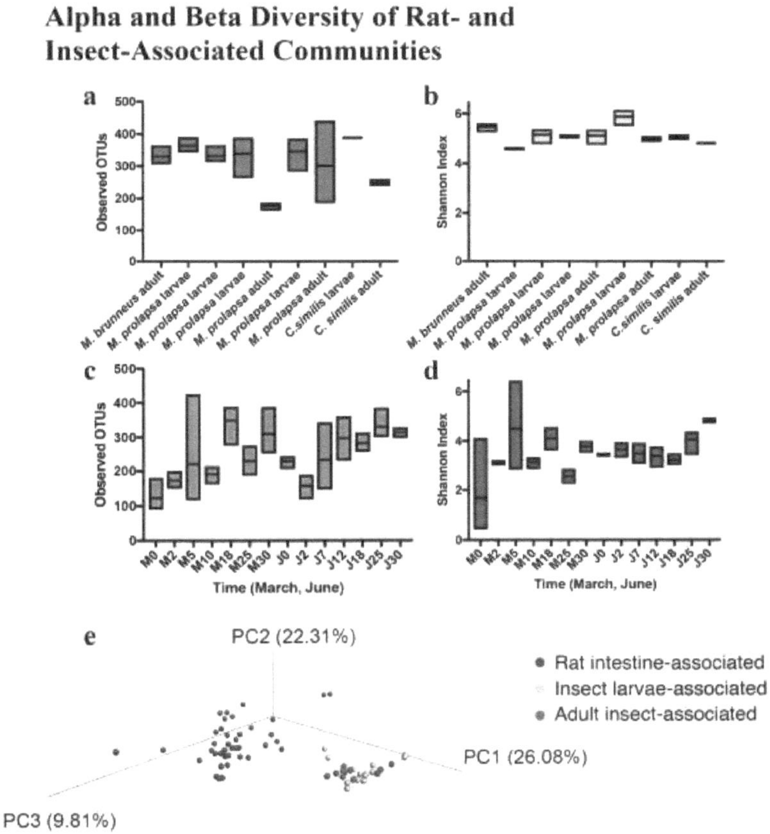

Figure 28: Alpha diversity in insect-associated and rat intestine-associated microbiomes is indicated by the abundance of operational taxonomic units (OTUs) and Shannon's Diversity Index (a, b, c, d). Beta diversity in the decomposition microbiome is evaluated using weighted UniFrac distances (e) [327].

Decomposition dynamics

The depositional setting includes environmental factors such as temperature and soil chemistry, which can impact the decomposition process. The presence of oxygen in the soil, determined by soil type, can affect the rate of decomposition and the microbial community structure. Therefore, distinguishing between buried and exposed taphonomic studies is crucial, particularly in the realm of estimating postmortem interval, if buried remains are subjected to different temperature and environmental conditions from direct soil contact. Temperature is a key variable that influences decomposition, with the most favorable range for soft tissue decomposition falling between 20°C and 40°C. In the current study, temperature played a significant role from two perspectives. Firstly, lower temperatures observed in the early spring experiment (March) hindered the putrefaction process. During this period, soil and air temperatures fluctuated between 7.28°C–10.76°C and 3.96°C–16.3°C, respectively, resulting in incomplete carcass decomposition by the end of day 30 [328]. Secondly, the stages and their transitions were not clearly differentiated, and the lower temperature thresholds could have prevented insect species presence and activity, considering that temperatures above 10 °C and 15 °C are optimum for their activity83. Unlike March, June was characterized by a soil and air temperature of 16.75 °C–25.37 °C and 15.8 °C–28.13 °C, respectively. The separate decomposition stages were observed entirely up to the beginning of skeletonization. It is of note that the minimum soil temperatures in both experimental periods were higher than the air temperatures, with the highest values observed above ground (Figure 29) [329].

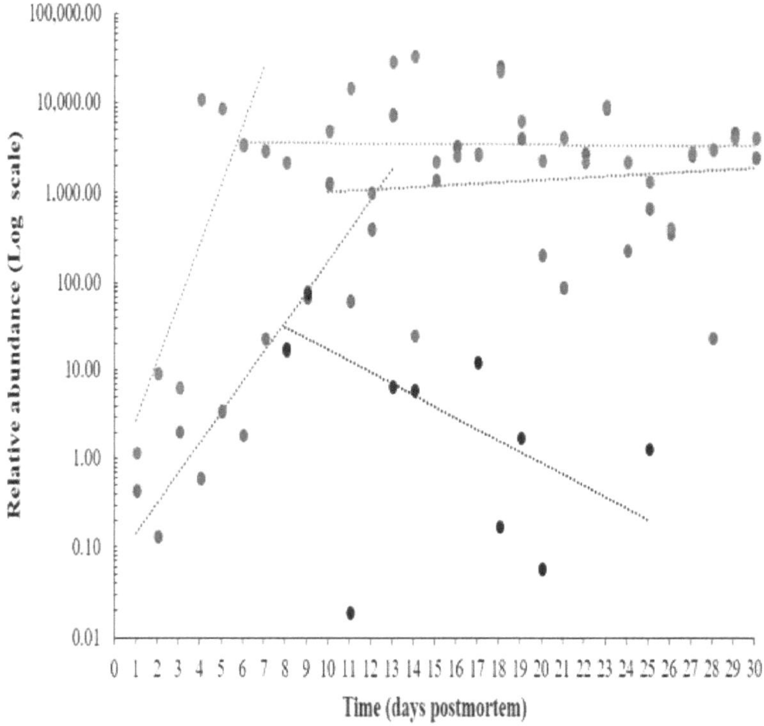

Figure 29: Relative abundance of Firmicutes species as a function of the postmortem time. *Enterococcus faecalis* (March – red; June – green), *Clostridium paraputrificum* (March – black). The logarithmic scale represents the number of bacterial cells. Temperature doesn't fluctuate very much in soil, lower thresholds can prevent, inhibit, or stop decomposition, similar to what was observed during March of the current study [327]

Temperature, among other factors, plays a crucial role in determining the postmortem interval. Obtaining meteorological data for outdoor conditions is relatively straightforward through weather stations, but procuring underground data poses challenges. Fortunately, temperature fluctuations are less pronounced below-ground compared to above-ground conditions, with the experiment showing minimal differences between air and soil temperature, ranging from 0.04 °C to 5 °C in March and 2.89 °C in June. Previous research has also noted the close correlation between air and soil temperature readings. In forensic investigations, air temperature readings can serve as a substitute when soil temperature data is unavailable for estimating the postmortem interval. However, caution is warranted in interpreting these results due to their variability and dependence on climate and soil characteristics. Moreover, temperature can impact the proliferation and diversity of bacteria. Studies have demonstrated that lower temperatures can impede microbial activity, leading to a slower rate of decomposition and body preservation. On the other hand, temperatures ranging from 10 °C to 30 °C can enhance microbial activity, particularly in the production of enzymes responsible for breaking down organic matter [258].

Although it cannot directly compare the findings from bacterial analysis to those of an exposed carcass, it is important to note that the soil temperature and ambient temperature did not show significant differences, with an average variance of only 5 °C. This demonstrates that temperature alone may not have been the sole factor influencing the microbial community. Additionally, the soil chemistry of the environment where decomposition occurred, such as the pH levels, could have impacted the structure of the microbial community over time. Previous studies have suggested that highly alkaline soils may hinder the survival of bacterial species involved in decomposition, but in the study, the soil was only slightly alkaline (reaching a maximum pH of 8.84 in March), and therefore did not appear to influence changes in bacterial abundance, as indicated by the results of Pearson's correlation analysis. It has been suggested that slightly alkaline soils can actually promote the growth of bacteria involved in decomposition. It was observed that an overall increase in pH levels from the initial stages of decomposition in March to the start of active decay in June. This pattern differs from observations made by Carter and Tibbett, who found high soil alkalinity during the early stages, followed by a decrease in pH (4.7) [329]. Another study conducted by Carter and colleagues on juvenile rat specimens showed an increase in soil pH levels up to 8.0 in all grave soils [330]. Wilson and collaborators noted a significant rise in pH levels during the decomposition of pig carcasses at depths of 0.3 and 0.6 cm. It is important to consider the soil type and moisture levels in interpreting these findings, as they could influence the similarities or differences observed in various studies, including factors such as oxygen content [331].

Insect dynamics on buried rat carcasses

The deposition environment may also include biological elements such as colonizing insects and microbial communities. The presence of Diptera and Coleoptera specimens was documented during the June experimental phase, beginning on the ninth day after burial, at a temperature of 18.67 °C. The research on *M. prolapsa* aligns largely with previous studies regarding the depth at which this species can colonize and its most active periods. Specifically, *M. prolapsa* demonstrated an ability to colonize at a depth of 40 cm, a behaviour also observed in the experiment conducted by Gunn and Bird, even in the presence of bait at the soil surface [333].

The research indicated that adult Muscidae were able to colonize buried remains within 30 minutes when enclosed, while we observed colonization occurring after 9 days. Although *M. prolapsa* was observed colonizing buried remains in both scenarios, the conditions of exposure could have influenced the timing of colonization, as the study did not involve enclosing or restricting insect movement. A previous study utilizing rat carcasses buried at depths ranging from 10 to 40 cm found that *M. prolapsa* colonized and eventually pupariated after 8 to 12 days, similar to other observations of a pupation period of 10 days with rats buried at 40 cm. Unlike the findings of Gunn and Bird, who observed *M. prolapsa* puparia in the top 4 cm of soil, which only collected *M. prolapsa* puparia at a depth of 40 cm. Furthermore, research conducted in the UK showed that *M. prolapsa* exhibited activity during the months of June to August, which aligns with the observations in Romania during the month of June. Typically, *M. prolapsa* is active during the warmer months of the year in regions with a temperate climate. While the activity period in other experiments varied, spanning from early spring to late autumn, it was generally agreed upon that June and July were the primary peak months of activity for this species [334 - 336].

During the course of this experiment, the aforementioned behavior was consistently documented, which may be expected considering the widespread distribution of this species in Eastern Europe and the moderate climate conditions found in Romania. An additional species from the Muscidae family, known as *M. levida*, was recognized in both the preceding and current investigations, albeit only observed briefly. In general, *M. prolapsa* stands out as a valuable marker for estimating the time since death of buried remains, owing to its capability to locate and inhabit buried remains, its prevalence in such environments, and its broad distribution across different regions [337].

During the June experiment, the second family of Diptera identified was Phoridae. The species in this family are typically found in buried environments, with observations ranging from 10 cm to 2 m deep (coffin depth). Previous experiments have primarily observed, collected, and identified Conicera species within this family [336- 338]. The data depicts the presence of two species from the Phoridae family, namely *Conicera similis* and *Megaselia rufipes*, in which *Conicera* was found to be more prevalent and consistently observed. In this particular case, adult *C. similis* were spotted after 9 days post-burial, contrasting with previous studies that noted the presence of *Conicera* sp. after 4 days post-burial at a depth of 25–50 cm. The adults and larvae of *M. rufipes* were collected during days 11–16, corresponding to the middle and end of the active decomposition phase, aligning with observations made for the sister species M. scalaris Loew 186685 on buried pig carcasses at a depth of 60 cm. Staphylinidae representatives from the *Coleoptera* order exhibit predatory behaviour towards immature dipterans, often appearing during the final stages of decomposition.

Although this family is not as dominant in soil, it is frequently seen in burial settings. While previous studies have highlighted the presence of *Philonthus* sp. as a key species found in buried carcasses, the observation only revealed *M. brunneus* towards the conclusion of the advanced decomposition phase. However, coleopteran species are not utilized for estimating postmortem intervals and are not considered relevant for forensic investigations. Their presence is merely acknowledged due to their predatory behaviour, which can impact dipteran larval populations and the overall decomposer community [339-341].

Insect microbiome

In order to gain a clearer insight into the bacterial populations linked to necrophagous insect adults and larvae, three specific species were examined: *M. brunneus*, *M. prolapsa*, and *C. similis*. Detailed examination of *C. similis* has already been addressed in a prior publication and will not be delved into here. A study conducted previously explored the bacterial communities associated with insects as they progress through the development stages of two species of Calliphoridae (Lucilia sericata Meigen, 1826 and Lucilia cuprina Wiedemann, 1830) [342].

Despite focusing on a different family of necrophagous Diptera in their investigation, the dominant phyla identified were Proteobacteria and Firmicutes, consistent with current observations of Diptera and recent experiments involving other Calliphoridae species. In contrast to earlier research, the present study revealed *Actinobacteria* as a prevalent phylum, with relative abundances ranging from 15 to 25% across various insect taxa. This discrepancy could be attributed to differences in insect species as well as variations between laboratory and field experiments, where samples in other studies had direct contact with the soil. Across different necrophagous insect families, species within the genera *Ignatzshineria*, *Proteus*, and *Clostridium* were frequently encountered. Previous studies have demonstrated that certain bacterial taxa are closely associated with insect species, sometimes producing enzymes that aid in tissue decomposition during the decomposition process [331].

Carcass microbiome

Numerous research inquiries have delved into the microbial composition during decomposition. Collectively, these inquiries reveal a decline in microbial variety parallel to diminishing nutrients until skeletonization, a trend which was not evident in the current data as diversity-maintained variability yet stability over time. Nonetheless, a significant portion of these studies conducted experiments involving exposed carcasses of mice, humans, or swine [343- 347].

The appearance of a decomposing carcass may vary due to factors such as the environment in which it is deposited and the types of organisms responsible for breaking it down, both of which can influence the decomposition rate and the estimation of the post-mortem interval. The research aligns with past studies on decomposition, particularly in relation to changes in the Firmicutes and *Proteobacteria* phyla within the intestines and abdominal cavities. However, unlike these previous studies, the findings revealed a reduced presence of Bacteroidetes and an increased prevalence of *Actinobacteria*. Previous research has indicated that Bacteroidetes are less common in the gut microbiomes of living rats compared to humans, potentially explaining initial disparities in decomposition processes between studies. *Actinobacteria* are typically found in soil environments, raising the possibility that these bacteria were associated with the buried rat carcasses, even though the specific characteristics of the soil microbial communities were not examined in this particular study [348, 349]. It should be emphasized that the absence of an exposed carcass as a burial control does not allow for the resolution of differences between insect or microbial community dynamics of buried or exposed remains, but instead offers a descriptive observation of buried rat carcasses. During the initial decomposition stages in June, Firmicutes was the most prevalent phylum, consistent with previous research on decomposed rat carcasses. Conversely, in March, *Proteobacteria* was the predominant phylum. These variations in phylum abundance could be influenced by temperature, as Firmicutes thrived in higher temperatures according to past studies and the current experiment, whereas *Proteobacteria* flourished amidst lower temperatures typically experienced in March. Furthermore, it is crucial to recognize that the microbial community structure and composition within mammalian hosts display both interspecies and intraspecies variability, similar to observations in humans. This underscores an increasingly significant aspect for future decomposition studies, as the microbial communities within the host, the surrounding environment, and the colonizers and scavengers may collectively impact the community structure and dynamics, thereby influencing the estimation of the postmortem interval [351].

In search of bacterial PMI biomarkers

In the months of March and June, a quantitative analysis was conducted on two Firmicutes taxa, *Enterococcus faecalis* and *Clostridium paraputrificum*, during the decomposition process of buried rat carcasses. The study marked the initial examination of these taxa in such a context. *Enterococcus faecalis* is a recognized commensal bacterial species found in the gastrointestinal tract of both humans and non-human mammals. This species has the potential to become an opportunistic pathogen, causing nosocomial infections, and is commonly present in small numbers in the healthy human small intestine, where it primarily survives through fermentation of unabsorbed sugars [352-357]. Furthermore, *Enterococcus faecalis* has the ability to thrive in extreme environmental conditions such as high salinity and pH levels, and can metabolize a variety of resources. The rapid increase in the relative abundance of this species during the bloating phase of decomposition can be attributed to its capacity to ferment glucose, metabolize carbohydrates, diamino acids, and glycerol, leading to microbial proliferation as the carcass is consumed. Although the initial abundance of *E. faecalis* varies depending on the season, the levels in March and June tend to converge as decomposition progresses. The rise in abundance of *E. faecalis* in June compared to March can be attributed to the difference in temperature, with the warmer summer months providing optimal conditions for the growth of this species. This aligns with the temperature range at which *E. faecalis* can thrive, from 10°C to 42°C, with 37°C being the ideal temperature [357, 358]. The potential utility of this species as a marker for estimating the post-mortem interval shows promise, given its probable presence in intestinal tissues. However, further investigation is necessary to test this hypothesis, as the makeup of bacterial communities can vary widely within and among mammalian gastrointestinal tracts, potentially influenced by the circumstances of death. The quantitative analysis of *C. paraputrificum* from the same samples revealed its initial appearance at the transition from partial bloating to active decay. Unlike *E. faecalis*, this taxon is rarely associated with human infections and its clinical significance is not well understood. Previous studies on quantifying Clostridiales involved in decomposition have only been conducted at the family level, without focusing on specific species. This bacterium is recognized to be strictly anaerobic, chitinolytic, Gram-positive, and mesophilic, producing acetic and propionic acids, along with significant amounts of gas through the fermentation process [359-362]. Despite the fact that this particular method of metabolism appears to align with the bloating and active decomposition process resulting in the production of significant amounts of gas by microbial biomass, the specific taxon responsible was not consistently detected, and a definitive conclusion could not be reached. Given the limited research on this taxon and the absence of information regarding its role in decomposition, further research is necessary. There are currently only a few studies that concentrate on quantifying bacteria associated with the decomposition process as potential indicators for estimating the postmortem interval, particularly those belonging to the phyla Firmicutes, *Actinobacteria*, and Bacteroidetes. The research revealed a significant increase in the relative abundance of *E. faecalis* (Firmicutes) by 3-4 orders of magnitude, whereas another study found that the relative abundance of other Firmicutes taxa (*Lactobacillus* spp.) decreased by three orders of magnitude. In general, these findings suggest that utilizing quantitative microbiome data may be a viable method for estimating the postmortem interval [363].

Nevertheless, it is important to anticipate variations in quantity due to the unique ante mortem microbiome composition present in each carcass.

Identifying common or "core" bacterial species and analyzing their respective levels before and after death could serve as valuable indicators for determining postmortem intervals. Integrating microbiology alongside entomology will enhance the understanding of the decomposition of buried carcasses by offering a comprehensive perspective on the decomposition process, which can be applied in forensic studies and inquiries [364].

Forensic Entomology

Forensic entomology encompasses various practices, ranging from examining pests in food products to investigating insect infestations in residential settings. Nonetheless, the most notable application of forensic entomology is in the realm of criminal investigations, particularly in instances of unexplained deaths. This field has a long history, dating back centuries. Remarkably, the earliest recorded use of forensic entomology to resolve a murder occurred in China in 1235. In contemporary times, insects are frequently utilized to determine the minimum post-mortem interval (PMI), more commonly referred to as the time of death. Among the most crucial insects for forensic entomologists in this regard are flies, with blow flies, belonging to the Calliphoridae family usually being the first to arrive at a corpse. Blow flies possess a highly developed sense of smell, enabling certain species to detect a deceased body from distances of up to 16 kilometres away. They are considered pivotal for estimating the PMI due to their rapid response time in reaching a body. In certain scenarios, blow flies have been observed to appear within a mere 10 minutes of a body becoming available for colonization (Figure 30) [365].

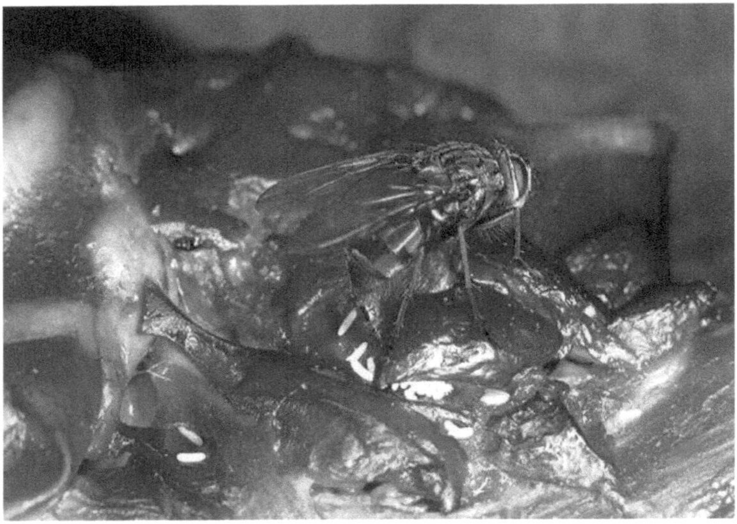

Figure 30: a blow fly laying its eggs on carrion[365]

Dr. Martin Hall, an expert in forensic entomology, has highlighted species within the family Calliphoridae as the optimal choice for determining a time of death. In a recent live stream discussion, he emphasized the inquisitive nature of these flies, noting that they are drawn to human remains and play a crucial role in the decomposition process. Blow flies, a common type in this family, possess the ability to lay numerous eggs on a corpse, with the larvae (maggots) proceeding to grow and develop through various stages known as instars. As they reach the pupation stage, the larvae encase themselves in a protective structure, undergoing a transformation into adult flies akin to the chrysalis phase of a butterfly's life cycle [366].

When analyzing the timeline of death, forensic entomologists must consider key factors such as the specific fly species involved, the developmental stage of the larvae, and the ambient temperature in which they have been developing. Warmer temperatures typically accelerate the growth and development of the larvae, affecting the overall estimation of the postmortem interval [366].

Studying human decomposition

Determining the time of death through insect activity is a complex process that is subject to various influencing factors. The rate at which flies go through their life cycle can be affected by different circumstances, such as the body being suspended or enclosed which can hinder maggot attachment and delay egg-laying by adult flies. In cases where bodies are discovered indoors, decomposition may occur at a different pace compared to bodies found outdoors. Moreover, the presence of narcotics in a deceased body can alter the development of maggots (Figure 31) [367].

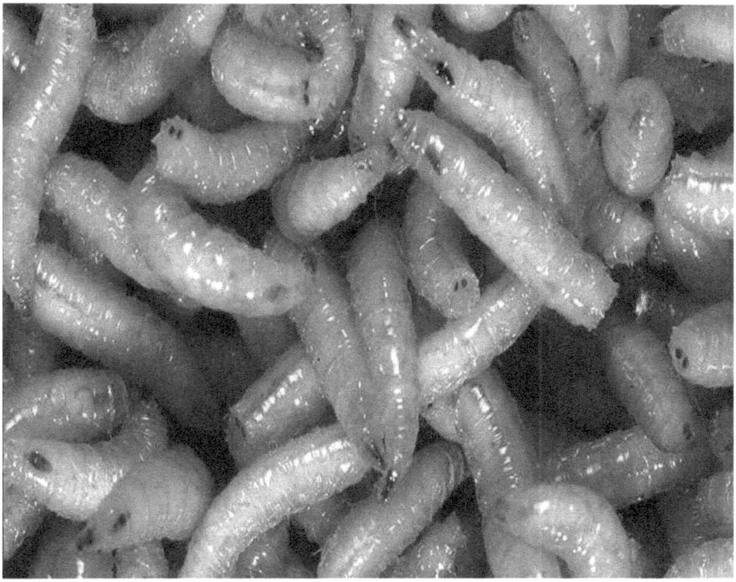

Figure 31: egg-laying by adult flies [367]

Numerous environmental variables possess the ability to significantly influence the growth and development of maggots. Therefore, it is imperative for forensic entomologists to possess a thorough comprehension of these factors when striving to establish a precise post-mortem interval. One of the ways scientists work to understand the impact of these and other factors on human decomposition is through 'body farms' - more formally known as human taphonomy facilities. The first was set up in 1981 in Tennessee, USA. These facilities are locations where donated cadavers are placed in various environments for detailed study. Researchers utilize these sites to educate themselves on distinguishing between deaths that occurred naturally and those that were brought about by unnatural factors [368].

Various climates play a significant role in the process of decomposition. For example, the decomposition process observed at a body farm in Michigan during the winter season would differ greatly from that of a body decomposing at a facility in Australia during the summer months. Although body farms have not yet been established in the United Kingdom, scientists in the country often examine the decomposition process using pigs as substitutes. Despite their value in forensic research, body farms encounter challenges such as regulatory hurdles and stigmatization as morbid institutions, leading to doubts surrounding their scientific merit [368].

Forensic entomology at the Museum

The scientists have collaborated with law enforcement in the examination of post-mortem intervals (PMIs) and have participated in research projects that have propelled the field of forensic entomology forward. For instance, the development process of blow flies like Calliphora vicina from egg to adult fly typically lasts around 19 days, with half of that period dedicated to the puparium stage. The puparia, being opaque, present a challenge for investigators in accurately determining the age of the insect found inside them at crime scenes. The opacity of fly pupae presents challenges when determining the age of the developing insect inside. However, advancements in technology now allow scientists to utilize micro-CT scanning to peer into the rigid outer shells of the pupae (Figure 32) [368].

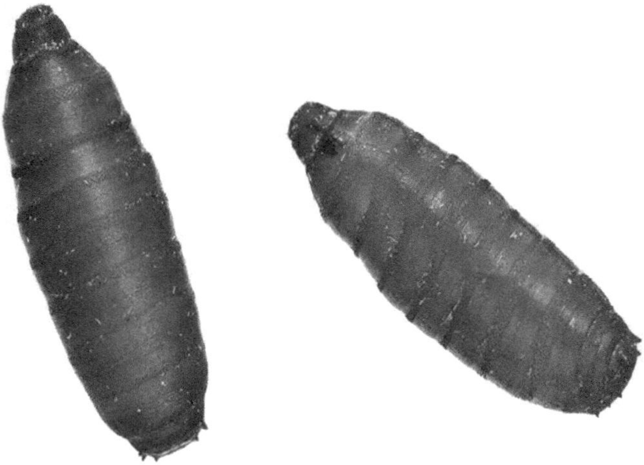

Figure 32: puparia fly [368]

In 2017, Martin articulated the importance of avoiding the dissection of puparia to preserve forensic evidence, emphasizing the need for non-invasive methods in forensic entomology research. The team of scientists opted for X-ray and micro-CT scanning to observe the internal changes in puparia throughout their development, noting the predictable alterations at specific temperatures [369].

Forensic entomology delves into the utilization of insect and arthropod studies in legal contexts, requiring a comprehensive understanding of biodiversity, biology, ecology, and behaviour to determine valuable information such as time of death, crime location, and sometimes cause of death. While the use of forensic insects in criminal investigations has a history of several decades, it has recently gained prominence as a distinct and sought-after field within forensic science. The accurate identification and analysis of regional insect species and their population patterns are crucial components in conducting effective medico-legal entomology for criminal cases [369].

The multifaceted nature of forensic entomology encompasses urban, stored products, and medico-legal aspects, with different insect groups colonizing corpses in specific patterns based on the stage of decomposition. The presence of certain insect species on a corpse aids in determining the level of decay, with the Calliphoridae family playing a pivotal role in estimating the time of death in cases where traditional methods fall short. Estimating the post-mortem interval relies on the development of maggots and the succession of entomofauna, with advancements in forensic toxicology, palynology, DNA analysis of insect species, and other innovative techniques contributing to the evolving landscape of forensic entomology, garnering substantial interest among criminal investigators and forensic experts alike [369].

Insects are commonly perceived as harmful organisms that negatively impact human health, agriculture, livestock, and various household materials. However, they also play a significant role in providing valuable commercial products such as honey, often referred to as liquid gold or the food of the gods, silk which is hailed as the supreme textile fiber, and lac which is utilized as sealing wax, cosmetics, and dyes. Moerover, about one-third of crop production is a result of insect pollination, highlighting their crucial ecological contribution [370].

The influence of insects in the realm of genetics is undeniably substantial and enduring. In addition, they serve as environmental cleansers by scavenging during decomposition processes. Notably, forensically important insects, functioning as scavengers, play a pivotal role in criminal investigations. When a deceased individual, whether human or wildlife, is discovered, forensic scientists typically inquire about the time of death, the cause, and the location of death. In instances involving decomposed or mutilated corpses, forensic entomology emerges as an indispensable tool for investigators, aiding in the procurement of crucial evidence [364].

Many researchers have utilized forensic entomology to estimate postmortem intervals in cases of human fatalities. Consequently, forensic entomology has emerged as a distinct and recognized sector of forensic science, with the acceptance of entomological evidence in legal proceedings expanding worldwide. [365].

Forensic Entomology can be characterized as the examination of insect species found on deceased individuals in criminal cases presented in court. Numerous experts in this field assert that crucial insect evidence remains highly reliable, precise, and occasionally the sole method for determining the time elapsed since death, even after a span of 72 hours [366- 369].

Traditionally, the calculation of the time elapsed since death has relied on evaluating the external features of cadavers, taking into account elements like temperature, body cooling, changes in the eyes, skin tone, muscle relaxation, rigor mortis, and post-mortem lividity. In cases where these indicators are not visible due to the decomposition or damage of the bodies, forensic entomology serves as a crucial form of evidence, enabling the determination of the post-mortem interval (PMI) through the analysis of insect colonization patterns [370, 371].

The use of legal entomofauna analysis in forensic investigations has gained increased acknowledgement due to the fact that insects are typically the initial organisms to colonize a decomposing body or a crime scene in a distinct sequence known as a succession wave. This succession wave is characterized by the predictable arrival patterns of various insect species, which can vary based on factors such as geographical location, season, and habitat. By examining the developmental stages and metamorphosis of these insects, experts can accurately determine the postmortem interval and potential manner of death [372- 378].

The expertise of a forensic entomologist can provide valuable information to assist investigative agencies in unraveling potential civil and criminal cases. Insects have long been recognized as reliable forensic indicators, with a history dating back to the 13th century. The earliest documented use of insects as tools for crime detection occurred in China in 1235 during a murder investigation detailed in Sung Tzu's medico-legal text, "The Washing Away of Wrongs: A Training Manual on Investigating Death." In this case, the sudden appearance of various blowflies on a specific sickle led to a murderer confessing to the killing of a fellow farm worker with the same weapon. A significant milestone in the establishment of medico-legal entomology as a credible forensic tool was the involvement of Dr. Bergeret in a case involving the murder of a newborn infant.

Dr. Bergeret, renowned as one of the pioneer forensic entomologists, discovered a mummified infant body hidden in a chimney during the investigation. Through the examination of insect larvae, specifically Sarcophaga carnaria and various moths, Dr. Bergeret was able to make informed assessments and determine that the infant had been concealed in 1848, with moth infestation occurring in 1849 [379].

In 1894, Megnin released a publication titled "La faune des corpses," presenting eight hypotheses regarding the progression of colonization by insects on cadavers left in the open, as well as two theories concerning buried corpses. His research concentrated on the characteristics of wing venation, posterior spiracles, and the general anatomy of insects for the purpose of categorization. Megnin's contributions to forensic entomology were widely acclaimed [375].

Types of Forensic Entomology

Entomology originates from the combination of the two ancient Greek terms 'entomon' (meaning insect) and 'logia' (meaning study), signifying the systematic examination of insects. Forensic entomology pertains to any aspect of the study of insects and their arthropod counterparts that has implications in legal contexts. This specialized field, forensic entomology, involves the analysis of insects found on a deceased human or protected animal to establish the time elapsed since death and address other pertinent investigative questions. Forensic entomology is inextricably linked with the broader scientific fields of medical entomology, forensic palynology, wildlife forensic entomology, taxonomy, and forensic pathology. Lord and Stevenson categorized forensic entomology into three primary divisions: [373]

1. Urban entomology: Legal proceedings involving insects and related animals which affect man-made structures and other aspects of the human environment.

2. Stored products entomology: Proceedings involving insects infesting stored commodities such as cereals and other household products.

3. Medico-legal entomology: Sometimes termed as "forensic medical entomology", and in reality should be termed as "medico criminal entomology" (because it focuses on violent or heinous crimes), relates primarily to:

- Determine the time since death (postmortem interval).
- Site /location/place of death (primary and secondary crime site).
- Manner/ mode of death [368].
- Cases of death especially with the help of forensic entomo-toxicology.
- Negligence of old age persons.
- Possible criminal acts or misuse of insects [380].

Decomposition of Human corpse and entomofauna association

After the death of an organism, there is a process known as autolysis where cells, tissues, and organs begin to degrade due to the action of biocatalysts. This leads to the decomposition of the corpse. Specifically in the gastrointestinal tract, bacteria initiate the breakdown of soft tissues, causing internal organs to liquefy and release gases such as carbon dioxide, methane, hydrogen sulfide, ammonia, sulfur dioxide, and hydrogen [381]. Forensically significant insects are drawn to volatile organic compounds called **apenumones**, emitted by the decaying body. This is a crucial factor in determining the postmortem interval as the behaviour of forensic insects is largely influenced by the unique substances released during the later stages of decomposition [382]. Generally, four categories of forensic entomofauna can be found on the decomposing corpse [369]:

- **First category:** Nacrophagous species, feeding on the corpse.
- **Second category:** Predators or parasites' species, feeding on the nacrophagous species.
- **Third category:** Omnivorous species, feeding on corpses and other arthropods (wasps, ants, and coleopterans).
- **Fourth category:** Springtails and spiders use corpses as an extension of their sweet homes.

Five decomposing stages based on the external physical appearance of a human corpse and internal temperature suggested by Tullis and Goff [19] are as follows:

1. Fresh stage

This marks the commencement of decomposition. During this phase, cellular breakdown takes place, forensic entomofauna presence is detected, there is no egg-laying, and it typically spans a duration of 24 to 48 hours.

2. Bloated stage

In this stage, putrefaction starts and gases accumulate in the body. There is a massive attendance of insects and oviposition is found. The duration of this stage is 2-7 days (seasons and habitats should also be considered).

3. Active decay stage/ decay stage

During this phase, the body begins to decay as a result of the release of gases. The abdominal walls become permeated, leading to deflation and bloating of the corpse. Signs of this stage include elevated internal temperature, a strong odour, reduction in the body weight of the deceased, and the transformation of third instar larvae into the pupal stage. The duration of this stage typically lasts between 5 to 13 days.

4. Advanced decay stage/ post decay

During this phase of larval growth, the insect consumes remaining skeletal and hard tissue remnants, as well as proteins. A notable aspect of this stage is the presence of a significant amount of moist, sticky matter known as decay by-products (BOD's), which serves as a breeding ground for the developmental processes of insects. The duration of this particular stage typically ranges from 10 to 23 days [381].

5. Dry remains stage/ Skeletonized stage

This marks the ultimate phase of decomposition of the body. The population of insects is decreasing, and the Biological Oxygen Demand is reduced to its lowest level during this stage. The duration of this phase typically ranges from 18 to 90 days [383].

Insects as a forensic indicator in crime investigation

Various inquiries that arise during criminal investigations and forensic examinations of a crime scene or deceased body, including determining the time of death, cause of death, and location of death, can be efficiently addressed through the study and observation of the succession patterns of forensic insects, as well as the age, weight, length, and developmental stages of maggots. The presence of forensic insects on a decaying body in different environments serves as valuable forensic evidence, as these insects colonize the body in a specific order [376].

The expected sequence of stages in the life cycle of insects displays variability based on factors such as biological influences, geographical locations, seasonal changes, and specific habitats. The growth rates and developmental progress of insects from larvae to adults serve as valuable tools in determining with precision the post-mortem interval and the manner of death [378].

Major forensic entomofauna

- **Calliphoridae (Blow flies)** which known as the first visitors to crime scenes:

1) **Blue bottle flies**: *Calliphora vomitoria, Calliphora livida, Calliphora hilli* etc.
2) **Green bottle flies**: *Chryosomya rufifacies, Chryosomya megacephala, Lucilia sericata, Lucilia cuprina, Lucilia illustris* etc.
3) **Black blow flies**: *Phormia regina*

- ***Sarcophagidae (Flesh flies)***: *Sarcophaga ruficornis, Sarcophaga pregrina, Sarcophaga albiceps, Sarcophaga africa, Sarcophaga caerulescens, Sarcophaga argyrostoma, Sarcophaga dux* etc.

- ***Muscidae (House flies)*:** *Musca domestica, Musca sorbens, Stomoxys calcitrans* etc.
- ***Piophilidae (Cheese flies)*:** *Piophila casei*
- ***Phoridae (Coffin flies)*:** *Conicera tibialis, Megaselia scalaris* etc.
- ***Staphylinidae (Rove beetles):*** *Staphylinidae lameere, Bryocharis analis, Tanygnathu sterminalis* etc.
- ***Silphidae (Carrion beetles):*** *Nicrophorus vespilloides, Nicrophorus nepalensis* etc.
- ***Cleridae (Checkered beetles):*** *Necrobia rufipes, Korynete scaeruleus* etc.
- ***Dermestidae (Skin/ hide beetles)*:** *Dermestes lardarius, Dermeste sater, Dermeste smaculatus* etc.

Dipteran insect shows complete metamorphosis

The typical life cycle of an insect is passed in the following stages: [383]

1. **Adult insects (flies) laid eggs:** an adult female fly is in search of a suitable location to deposit her eggs. Traditional bodily openings like the mouth, nostrils, anus, eyes, and wounds are frequently identified as ideal spots for egg-laying on a deceased body.

2. **Hatching of Eggs:** in the majority of species, eggs measure between 1 to 2 millimeters in length and commonly require a period of 1 to 2 days before hatching occurs.

3. **First instar larvae:** after the eggs have hatched, they transform into the initial stage of development known as first instar larvae, commonly referred to as maggots. These maggots consume the semi-liquid bodily fluids by releasing various biocatalysts or enzymes to break down the protein in their environment. As they feed, the maggots exhibit signs of growth, and within a few days, they undergo their first molting process wherein they shed their initial exoskeleton.

4. **Second instar larvae:** after the initial molting process, maggots progress to the second stage known as second instar larvae. As the enzymes continue to break down body tissues, they feed on the resulting decomposed materials and undergo growth in size, length, and weight. Upon reaching maturity, the second instar larvae undergo a second exoskeleton molt.

5. **Third instar larvae:** after undergoing their second moult, the larvae transition into third instar larvae. During this stage, the maggots cease feeding and enter a phase of pupation where they encase themselves in soft soil.

6. **Prepupa:** the mature larvae of insects, known as prepupae, begin to decrease in size and develop a slightly hardened exterior.

7. **Pupa:** the final exoskeleton does not disintegrate, rather it undergoes a process of hardening and transitions from a light brown color to a darker shade of brown before ultimately turning black.
8. **Empty puparium:** after the emergence of adult insects empty puparia are left.

Identification of larval instars

Various morphological characteristics are utilized in the identification and distinction of larval instars: [380]

• The total number of larval segments (11/12) can be distinguished, with the first or cephalic segment, which can be retracted into the second, being referred to as pseudocephalon.

• Discrimination between families can be achieved by observing unique arrangements of posterior spiracles within the Calliphoridae, Sarcophagidae, and Muscidae.

• Three primary taxonomic identification features of larval stages include the cephalopharyngeal skeleton, anterior and posterior spiracles.

• The cephalopharyngeal skeleton of second instar larvae is deeply pigmented and lacks an accessory sclerite beneath the mouth hook, whereas in third instar larvae, the cephalopharyngeal skeleton is heavily pigmented and an accessory sclerite is present beneath the hook region.

• Second-instar and third-instar larvae exhibit 8-9 papillae on each anterior spiracle, arranged in a line pattern that varies among species.

• The posterior spiracles of second instar larvae contain two spiracular slits without peritreme thickening, distinguishing them from the third instar larvae which have three slits per posterior spiracle.

• Only the last trunk segment mid-dorsally displays a pair of D-shaped posterior spiracles in first instar larvae, serving as external openings for body tracheae for respiration.

• Second and third instar larvae possess fan-shaped anterior spiracles dorsally on the thorax, aiding in respiration.

• Second and third-instar larvae can be differentiated by factors such as weight, length, and color.

• Discrepancies exist in the degree of sclerotization of specific parts of the cephaloskeleton, as well as the posterior spiracular peritreme.

• The shape of posterior spiracular slits is a key distinguishing feature.

• The overall shape of anterior spiracles, arrangement of their lobes, distribution, and shape of spines or warts on the inner band area of segments are significant for differentiation.

• Utilizing stereo zoom microscope (50X) and binocular microscope aids in the identification and differentiation of various stages.

Evidential value of forensic entomology in the court of law

The utilization of evidence derived from forensic entomology holds significant judicial value and has the potential to impact the trajectory of criminal investigations and legal proceedings in various ways. The oral and written accounts related to forensic arthropods can serve as an invaluable tool in investigations, providing a comprehensive analysis of relevant circumstances. Additionally, forensic entomofauna evidence may uncover critical aspects during the investigative process, shedding light on the truth [381].

Scientific insights gleaned from insect evidence can serve to support other forms of evidence, both tangible and testimonial. For entomological evidence to have a meaningful influence on legal outcomes, it must be introduced and considered within the framework of court proceedings. The evaluation of forensic insect evidence typically falls under the purview of session courts, High courts, the Supreme Court of India, and other judicial bodies, classified as expert testimony of a scientific nature [382].

In essence, the analysis of entomological data necessitates the expertise of individuals qualified to provide an informed perspective on how such evidence aligns with the specifics of a given case. The presentation of expert testimony is subject to the regulations outlined in state and central rules of evidence, or equivalent legal frameworks present in various jurisdictions [383].

Insects' collection, entomological preservation methods, simulation and rearing

The insect collection and their preservation methods are as follows: [384]

- **Collections of adult flies:** the capture of airborne arthropods for analysis, whether at artificial locations or authentic crime scenes, can be achieved utilizing aerial netting.
- **Collections of eggs and larval stages:** insect egg collections are typically conducted using a delicate paintbrush, and it is recommended to aim for an average sample size ranging from 50 to 100 eggs. Larval stages and pupae can be retrieved using gentle nose forceps or a disposable spoon.
- **Preservation:** collected specimens should be preserved in 70% ethanol.
- **Drying, pinning and taxonomic labeling:** all specimens gathered must be transported to the laboratory for the process of drying, labeling, and identification. Initially, the specimens are stored at room temperature before being placed in a desiccator box for thorough drying. Subsequently, they are pinned to aid in taxonomic identification.
- **Microscopy:** the examination of microscopic images of every life stage of insects should be conducted using a high-resolution stereo-zoom microscope or Scanning Electron Microscopy (SEM).
- **Environmental conditions:** the climatic conditions at the crime scene, such as temperature, humidity, and precipitation, should be documented. This information can be readily acquired from the closest Government Regional Meteorological Center.
- **Simulation and rearing:** Carcasses ought to be positioned in varying geological environments and different seasons, either on a white tray of

uniform dimensions or inside a standard-sized wooden coffin. Throughout the research period, the tray should be shielded by a standard-sized iron enclosure secured with chicken wire and stones to prevent disruption by domestic or wild animals. Plastic pots and wide-mouth bottles, with socks stretched over the openings, are employed for the purpose of rearing animals.

Recent advances in forensic entomology

Entomo-toxicology

Entomo-toxicology is the scientific examination of identifying poisons, toxins, or medications from various stages of insect development. Analysis of insect evidence gathered from crime scenes is crucial in determining the cause of death resulting from poisoning. Insects that have fed on the deceased body can provide valuable insight into the presence of toxic substances or drugs in the individual's tissues prior to death. In cases where dead bodies are highly decomposed or mutilated, rendering important organs or tissues destroyed, insects and their remains such as empty pupal cases or deceased insects can offer essential entomo-toxicological information [383].

Furthermore, forensic insects can be utilized to detect the presence of illicit drugs. Research by J C Beyer in 1980 has demonstrated that the use of arthropods in a deceased body or crime scene investigation can establish if toxins were within the individual's body at the time of death [384]. Forensic Entomo-toxicology has emerged as a new sub-branch of forensic entomology. J.C. Beyer, considered the pioneer in this field, is often referred to as the father of entomo-toxicology due to his significant contributions. In a notable criminal case involving the discovery of a young girl's corpse fourteen days post-mortem, Beyer successfully detected toxins, poisons, and drugs from entomological evidence, specifically maggots that had been feeding on the body. The advanced state of decomposition of the corpse rendered traditional toxicological analysis of organs and tissues impossible. By utilizing gas chromatography and thin-layer chromatography techniques, Beyer was able to identify Cochliomyia macellaria larvae and detect phenobarbital [384].

Additional scientific research, particularly from Western countries such as France, has further illustrated the role of insects in toxin detection. Investigations have revealed cases where drugs were not initially detected in body tissues even after a span of two months post-mortem, yet through liquid chromatography techniques, Kintz was able to identify trizopam in maggots. Some studies have suggested that maggot tissues may be more conducive for toxin detection compared to muscle tissues, and in certain instances, toxins can be identified during the diapauses phase of insects. The analysis of pupal cases and larval skins has also proven instrumental in detecting toxins long after death. Challenges arise when dealing with corpses in advanced stages of decay, as samples typically collected for toxicological examination, such as viscera, vomit, blood, and urine, may no longer be available [385].

In such circumstances, the entomological specimens (primarily flies and beetles) associated with the decedent can serve as a dependable alternative source for the analysis of various toxins, poisons, and drugs. Previous research has revealed the presence of a wide range of toxic compounds in the developmental stages of insects that feed on human remains, including substances like heroin, morphine, cocaine, triazolam, oxazepam, phenobarbital, methamphetamine, lead, and arsenic found in the tissues of maggots. Additionally, toxic substances can also be identified in the regurgitated matter and excrement of these insects, with their detection and analysis being conducted through sophisticated methods such as thin layer chromatography (TLC), high performance liquid chromatography (HPLC), gas chromatography-mass spectrometry (GC-MS), liquid chromatography-mass spectrometry (LC-MS), and Fourier-transform infrared spectroscopy (FTIR) [386- 391].

Wildlife Forensic Entomology

The significance of forensic entomology extends to cases involving wildlife crime investigations, such as illegal hunting, poaching, and trade regulated by The Wildlife Protection Act 1972, as it offers valuable information on factors including time since death, cause of death, and geographic location of the crime scene, similar to cases involving human fatalities. In 2010, two high-profile national cases involving the deaths of tiger cubs in Ranthambhore and a tiger in the Sariska National Park, a designated tiger reserve in Rajasthan, were successfully resolved through the collection and taxonomic identification of entomofauna found on the deceased animals, specifically the species of Chrysomya, commonly known as "hairy maggot blowflies." By studying the life cycle of these insects and taking into account various environmental factors such as season, temperature, rainfall, and relative humidity, the developmental and growth rates of larvae and pupae contributed to determining the postmortem intervals in both cases [392].

Instant insects' identification (DART-HRMS technology)

The University of Albany has recently utilized a sophisticated method known as direct analysis in real-time with high-resolution mass spectrometry (DART-HRMS) to examine Calliphoridae fly eggs. DART-HRMS, created by Dr. Chip Cody of JEOL, is an innovative ambient ionization mass spectrometry approach that allows for direct analysis of samples without time-consuming preparation steps and without sample destruction. This cutting-edge technique has shown the ability to quickly distinguish between different insect species by analyzing the amino acid profiles of their eggs, with certain amino acids such as alanine, isoleucine, and proline being common among species and others like glutamine and tryptophan being exclusive to specific species such as *P. regina*.

Molecular identification of insect species

The conventional techniques utilized in morphological identification are considered outdated and no longer relevant, particularly challenging for certain species and unreliable for immature life stages. These constraints have prompted scientists to transition towards a molecular approach utilizing Polymerase Chain Reaction-Restriction fragment length polymorphism (PCR-RFLP) of the mt-DNA. Mitochondrial COI and COII genes serve as suitable molecular markers due to the relatively high level of genetic diversity observed in this region. Given the challenges associated with identification based on physical characteristics, molecular identification techniques, such as DNA barcoding and PCR-RFLP, are preferred for their accuracy and efficiency. The application of molecular biology techniques in distinguishing insect species aids in the estimation of Post Mortem Interval (PMI). PCR-RFLP analysis is also utilized for identifying closely related species of forensic significance across different life stages, offering a simple, rapid, and cost-effective method for routine diagnostic purposes [392- 395].

Human DNA identification from larval gut portion

Recent advancements in the field have led to the development of methods for molecularly identifying insect species or detecting and differentiating human DNA present in the gut of insects that consume human remains. Maggots' digestive systems serve as a viable source for extracting DNA for the purpose of identifying both the insects themselves and the contents of their gut. In cases where obtaining DNA samples directly from the deceased individual is not feasible, such as when only skeletal remains are present or access to the body is restricted, it is possible to obtain a human short tandem repeat (STR) profile from maggots that have been feeding on decomposing tissue at an advanced stage of decay [32, 33].

Wide range of applications and multifarious approaches of forensic entomology

They are: [380]

1. Determination of the post-mortem interval is crucial in human forensic investigations.
2. The biogeographical location of death must be taken into consideration.
3. The displacement of the deceased's body plays a significant role in forensic analysis.
4. Identifying both the primary and secondary crime scenes is imperative.
5. The mode and manner of death are key factors in forensic evaluations. [368].
6. The cause of death is determined by the field of entomotoxicology.
7. There may have been a criminal exploitation of insects leading to the death.
8. Inadequate care for elderly individuals residing in their homes is a concerning issue.

9. The neglect of newborn babies in hospital settings is a matter of great importance.
10. Mysterious traffic accidents without clear causes are a significant area of concern.
11. Entomotoxicology refers to the identification of potential poisons or drugs through insect evidence.

12. The identification of human DNA through a larval gut portion is a groundbreaking technique.
13. Wildlife forensic entomological analysis and investigation play a crucial role in solving crimes.
14. The smuggling of narcotic plants in border regions presents a serious challenge for law enforcement.

Concepts, Procedures and Techniques Used by Forensic Entomologists and Proxies

While serving as an update, this review sets itself apart from other literature that primarily focuses on outlining the procedures and equipment needed by a seasoned forensic entomologist (FE) to perform an entomological examination of a crime scene. Emphasizing the importance of properly collecting and preserving insect evidence by individuals with the appropriate qualifications or under their supervision, the primary aim of this paper is to present a comprehensive guide on how less experienced personnel (who have received some training), such as crime scene technicians, forensic officers, and proxies, can gather and collect insect samples at a crime scene. This allows the FE to provide a more accurate estimation of the postmortem interval [398, 399].

Forensic science plays a vital role in the process of solving crimes by linking the investigation with legal proceedings. Currently, forensic science has branched out into various specialized areas, including forensic entomology, forensic toxicology, forensic anthropology, and forensic microbiology. These fields offer methods and guidelines for gathering and evaluating evidence related to crimes in order to recreate the precise conditions of a crime scene. This aids in establishing the occurrence of a crime and, ultimately, leads to legal action being taken [400-403].

The material evidence obtained from a crime scene is predominantly utilized to confirm the guilty parties while absolving any individuals of innocence, as well as elucidating the particulars of the crime including how, when, and where it occurred. The retrieved physical evidence can offer clues based on observation or necessitate sophisticated techniques for further analysis. For instance, a detailed examination of hair under a microscope could yield information regarding the age, gender, and ethnicity of an individual found at the scene of the crime. This could be followed by DNA analysis and spectroscopic analysis, providing insights into an individual's identity and the potential presence of explosive or drug residues [404, 405].

Forensic Entomology for Crime Scene Investigations

Forensic entomology is a field that utilizes insects and other arthropods to assist in the resolution of criminal and civil cases. It is typically categorized into three main subfields: urban entomology, stored product entomology, and medicolegal entomology. Urban entomology focuses on the impact of insects on building structures and medical myiasis. Stored product entomology is concerned with evaluating the risks of biosecurity breaches related to food contamination and environmental degradation. Lastly, medicolegal entomology employs insect-based evidence to investigate a range of criminal activities, including homicides, suspicious deaths, abuse of vulnerable individuals, hospital negligence, animal abuse, contraband trafficking, and wildlife poaching [406- 411].

Insects play a crucial role in forensic investigations by serving as biological markers to help determine the postmortem interval or time since death. Additionally, the presence and development of dipteran larvae in wounds caused by myiasis can offer valuable insights into the duration of neglect for various species, including humans, pets, and livestock. The underlying principles of using insects in such investigations involve estimating the postmortem interval by studying their development patterns based on temperature, as well as observing the sequential colonization of carcasses by different insect species [412, 413].

Flies, belonging to the Order Diptera, play a crucial role as the primary carrion arthropods in the estimation of postmortem interval. Their participation in the decomposition of corpses as early and long-lasting colonizers makes them a key focus in forensic entomology studies. Flies alternate between scavenging on decaying tissues and becoming prey for other carnivorous invertebrates like beetles and ants, as well as larger predators such as hyenas and vultures (Figure 33 a–d) [414- 416].

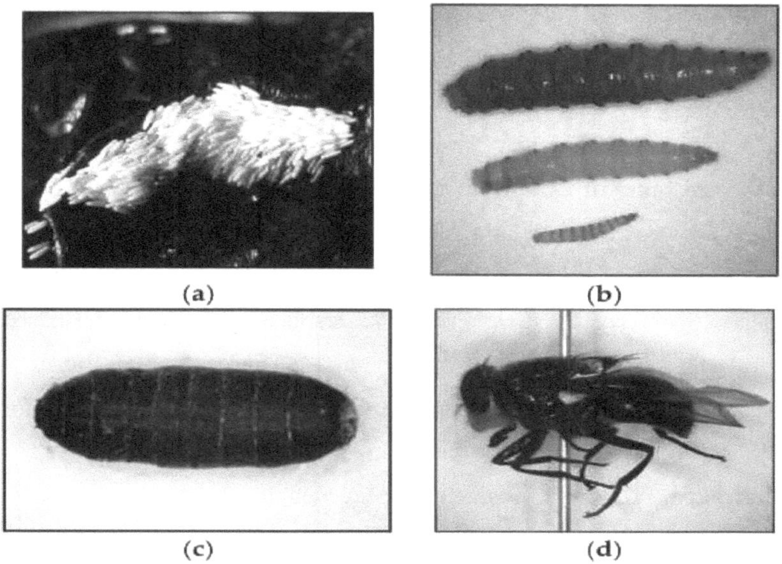

Figure 33: The life stages of a fly encompass various developmental phases. The data presented are sourced from Byrd and Tomberlin, 2020 [406]. The stages include: (a) Fly egg raft (individual egg size ranging from 1.2–2 mm). (b) Three larval instars (in increasing order; third, second, first instar with a size range of 2–23 mm). (c) Fly pupa (size range from 6–23 mm). (d) Adult fly (size range from 6–14 mm). Traditionally, the minimum post-mortem interval (minPMI) during the early stages of carcass decomposition (3–72 hours post-death) is determined using pathological techniques. However, beyond this time frame, fly eggs, larvae, and pupae serve as crucial indicators for establishing the age of a carcass. This is accomplished through three methods: (1) calculating accumulated degree day/hour units, (2) consulting life history tables, and (3) utilizing species-specific isomegalen/isomorphen curves. Furthermore, estimating the minPMI during advanced decomposition stages can involve examining the succession patterns of flies and other carrion-associated invertebrates, although this method is generally less precise [417- 421].

However, there are limitations to estimating the minimum PMI by examining fly development during advanced stages of decomposition. For instance, the fly larvae and puparia collected may not accurately represent the initial colonizers, as they may have already completed their life cycle. Typically, the expected order of fly attraction to carrion commences with the Calliphoridae family, followed by Sarcophagidae, Muscidae, Sphaeroceridae, Piophilidae, Fannidae, and Phoridae. In addition to flies, carcasses are also infested by beetles such as Staphylinidae, Scarabaeidae, Carabidae, Silphidae, Cleridae, and Dermestidae; moths like Pyralidae and Tineidae; and mites from Pterygosomatidae and Omentolaelapidae families, all of which can hold forensic significance [422- 425].

In addition, the order in which these invertebrates colonize a dead body may differ depending on a variety of external and internal factors, including alterations in the corpse's features (such as size, nutritional content, current level of decay, and presence of foreign substances), abiotic elements (such as temperature and moisture levels), and biotic aspects (including the surrounding terrestrial and aquatic environments) [423].

Estimating the minimum Post-Mortem Interval (minPMI) is a key aspect of forensic investigations. In some cases, entomological assessments can be conducted to determine the movement of carcasses from their initial crime scenes. This is based on the understanding that the insect species found on a carcass reflect the overall insect population of the surrounding environment, and any relocation of the carcass could alter this specific entomofauna. The decision to perform entomological assessments is influenced by the location of the crime scene and prevailing environmental factors. Furthermore, any disturbances to a carcass can result in the dispersal of fly larval clusters, particularly when they are densely aggregated. It is also possible to utilize the identified internal and external microbial compositions of larval clusters infesting carcasses to confirm the authenticity of a crime scene. This verification process involves comparing the microbial profiles of the larval clusters with those present at the crime scene to determine their similarity [426- 429].

Fly tissues have proven to be useful for identifying victims and determining the cause of death through the study of entomogenetics and entomotoxicology. This becomes especially significant in cases where the tissues and fluids of victims are not accessible for analysis due to factors such as tissue degradation caused by larval feeding, scavenging, or burning. By examining the contents of different parts of a fly's digestive system using DNA analysis, it is possible to uncover the identity of a victim. In addition, DNA can be extracted from flies at different stages of development to identify the species, by comparing their species-specific gene sequences with those in a genetic database. Furthermore, estimating the age of larvae and pupae based on gene expression provides another valuable molecular approach in forensic investigations [430- 435].

Previous research in entomotoxicology has demonstrated that tissues of flies can be utilized for the detection of various substances such as alcohol (specifically ethanol), drugs (including antidepressants, barbiturates, benzodiazepines, opioids, and phenothiazine), metals (such as thioridazine, antimony, barium, cadmium, lead, and mercury), and pesticides (like malathion and parathion). However, the accuracy and reliability of these genetic and toxicological analyses using flies are contingent on factors such as the species of fly, developmental stage, feeding habits, environmental factors, methods of insect sampling, the quantity of specimens collected, frequency of sampling, and techniques utilized for killing and preserving the insects [436- 438].

Forensic Entomologist: An Apprentice to an Expert

Analyzing the insect population at a crime scene is a multi-faceted process that involves collecting samples, identifying species, establishing relationships between species and their habitats, assessing growth stages and patterns, and studying insect behaviour in relation to changing climatic conditions. Becoming skilled in forensic entomology necessitates a strong foundation in entomology and ecology. In order to carry out these responsibilities, a forensic entomologist must possess an understanding of concepts like insect physiology, taxonomic and evolutionary connections, how insects adapt behaviorally to various environments, and the implications of these adaptations on human matters [438-440]. The training should be focused on specific topics that address the diagnostic characteristics and interrelationships of important insect groups in forensics. This specialized knowledge in forensic entomology can be obtained through undergraduate or postgraduate courses, as well as degree programs. In many countries, these formal qualifications are necessary for forensic entomologists to collaborate with local law enforcement agencies. It is important to emphasize that academic pursuits should be complemented by practical experience in crime scene investigation, adherence to protocols, and the ability to prepare expert witness statements and present evidence in court [441]. The cultivation of skills and experiences necessary for forensic entomology can be achieved through the implementation of simulated crime scene trials using surrogate human carcasses, notably swine. It is highly recommended to carry out these practical exercises under the guidance of a forensic entomologist with prior experience in real cases. Furthermore, a solid understanding of various related fields including molecular biology, microbiology, taphonomy, toxicology, pathology, and criminalistics is imperative for a comprehensive approach to forensic entomology [442- 445].

Forensic Entomology in Crime

Insects play a crucial role in the process of carcass decomposition. Flies and other arthropods are attracted to a carcass unless there are obstacles preventing their access. Once the food source (carcass) is depleted, the insects will depart. The colonization of insects on a carcass is heavily influenced by the climate based on the season and region, which includes factors such as temperature, humidity, and photoperiod. It also depends on the interactions within and between species, such as their feeding preferences and competition, as well as various habitat conditions such as terrestrial and aquatic environments, urban and rural settings, indoor and outdoor locations, and burial versus exposed conditions [445].

Moreover, secondary elements like the manner of demise, encompassing burning, poisoning, drowning, dismemberment, concealment, and hanging, along with the characteristics of the remains like age, dimensions, attire, and injuries, play a significant role in influencing the patterns of insect colonization and decomposition. The intricate nature of interactions between insects and remains presents a continuous challenge for Forensic Entomologist (FE) in carrying out their duties meticulously and accurately. Nevertheless, familiarity with the indigenous insect species, past involvement in insect-related forensic investigations, and the ability to integrate research findings into casework serve as the foundational elements necessary for an accurate estimation of the minimum post-mortem interval (minPMI) [446].

In addition to the intricate nature of carcass insects, a forensic entomologist must navigate various regulatory obstacles. These challenges include collaborating with other professionals at crime scenes, such as scientists and forensic agents, meeting strict deadlines for expert witness testimonies, and addressing conflicts in the courtroom [447, 448].

Progression and Standardisation in Forensic Entomology

Numerous seminal works by Mégnin (1894) and Payne (1965) illuminated the significance of insects in the process of carrion decomposition. These studies established the groundwork for the use of insects in forensic investigations. Mégnin (1894) was the first to put forth a formal definition and testable mechanism for insect succession on carrion, while Payne (1965) underscored the substantial role insects play in reducing carrion biomass during the initial stages of decomposition. Building upon these pioneering studies, numerous research projects have been conducted worldwide to develop keys for identifying carrion insects, document the succession of insects on carrion in varying environments and time frames, record the developmental stages of flies under field and laboratory conditions, and integrate forensic entomology with other disciplines such as genetics, toxicology, and microbiology. These findings have been utilized in various criminal investigations, published as case studies in books and scientific journals, presented at conferences, and occasionally featured in popular media. Together, these efforts have solidified forensic entomology as a reputable subfield within the realm of forensic science [449- 451].

The establishment of standardized entomological techniques for crime solving has enhanced the field of forensic entomology and has increased its recognition and credibility within law enforcement circles. Numerous significant research papers have been released, that analyze successional and developmental studies, thereby connecting academic research with practical application. As a result, there has been an enhancement in the guidelines and procedures utilized by forensic entomologists in actual criminal investigations [452- 455].

Several efforts have been undertaken to establish international guidelines that can aid a forensic examiner in conducting their duties in a methodical and systematic manner, both in field and laboratory settings [455]. The guidelines provided establish the fundamental protocols and necessary tools for an FE to carry out entomology-related duties at a crime scene and in a laboratory in order to determine precise estimates of the minimum postmortem interval. Nevertheless, these guidelines are flexible and subject to alteration (see Table 1) depending on the skill level and expertise of the practitioner, the resources available, and the specific conditions of the crime scene. The three levels of standards outlined (Gold, Silver, and Bronze) preserve the core procedures while offering alternative approaches to minimize any potential misunderstandings [456].

Occasionally, a forensic entomologist may not be available to attend a crime scene and perform the standard entomology procedures, leaving the task to a proxy with limited entomological expertise, such as a pathologist, crime scene technician, or law enforcement agent. These proxies rely on alternative methods known as Silver and Bronze standards, which reflect varying levels of knowledge and training in forensic entomology. While imperfect, these procedures can still provide enough information for a forensic entomologist to make a reasonable estimate of the minimum post-mortem interval (minPMI), although the evidence may not be admissible in court. Rather, it can help investigators narrow down a timeline for potential suspects. To aid in this process, reviewing a standard operating procedure for collecting insect evidence or observing an entomological crime scene application can be beneficial. It is important to regularly update these standards with new ideas and techniques. In the following section of this review, a crime scene technician or proxy may find helpful information on the responsibilities and requirements of a forensic entomologist when calculating the minPMI [456].

Table 1: A guide detailing three standards for forensic entomologists and their proxies to aid in collecting and preserving insect specimens [456]

Category	**Specific Entomological Aspect**	**Gold Standard**	**Silver Standard**	**Bronze Standard**
General	The person involved in sampling	Forensic entomologist (FE)	FE-trained police officer, medical examiner, or pathologist	The police officer or field technician (generally untrained)
	Number of times visiting a crime scene for and/or mortuary for entomology assessments	Initial visit followed by additional visits to gather climatic data and sift surrounding soil (especially when advanced decomposition is present)	Once	Once
	Clothing	Standard personal protection equipment [1] supplied by police/agency attending the crime scene	Standard personal protection equipment [1] supplied by police/agency overseeing crime scene or person acting in the FE role	Masks and gloves minimum standard personal protection equipment supplied by police/agency overseeing crime scene if present
Microclimatic data	Data collecting	Onsite data collection—	Nearest meteorological	Nearest meteorologica

Category	Specific Entomological Aspect	Gold Standard	Silver Standard	Bronze Standard
	equipment	infrared thermometer, temperature probe, temperature data logging device; Offsite data collection—nearest meteorological station	station data, analogue thermometer	1 station data
	Type of data collected at a crime scene	Ambient temperature, larval mass temperature, soil temperature, humidity, photoperiod, rainfall from nearest weather station	Ambient temperature, larval mass temperature), rainfall from nearest weather station	Ambient temperature, rainfall from the nearest weather station
	Duration of data collection	10–12 days at crime scene after discovery	Not applicable	Not applicable
Sampling of insects	Sampling equipment	Entomology kit [2], forceps (various sizes and types), spoons, artist paint brushes, insect net, sticky traps, containers (closed and	Disposable forceps, containers, preservatives (supplied by agency overseeing crime scene)	Disposable forceps, containers, and preservatives (supplied by the agency overseeing the

Category	Specific Entomological Aspect	Gold Standard	Silver Standard	Bronze Standard
		ventilated), refrigerated container (cooler or fridge) for transport		crime scene)
	Type and maturity stages of sampling insects	Eggs, larvae, full and empty puparia, adults of flies, and beetles	Eggs, larvae, full and empty puparia	Eggs, larvae, full and empty puparia
	Number of insects sampled	Depends on the location, access, and stage of life of the insects. The number of insects should cover the base of the container used	Depending on access, sample available insect material. Number of insects to cover the base of the container used. If possible, a minimum of 10 specimens chosen randomly	Depending on the access, sample available insect material (minimum 10 specimens chosen randomly)
	Labelling	Include date, time, case reference no., and type of specimen via indelible pen on the external label. Repeat in pencil and place this label inside	Include date, time, case reference no., and type of specimen via indelible pen on the external label. Repeat in pencil and	Include the date, time, case reference no., and type of specimen using a pencil on the label both outside and inside the

Category	Specific Entomological Aspect	Gold Standard	Silver Standard	Bronze Standard
		the container	place this label inside the container	container
Preservation of insects for morphological analyses and minPMI	Live insects (eggs/larvae /full puparia)	Retain a sample of insects (placed into ventilated containers) for later rearing. Place these in refrigeration or cooler. For eggs, add moist paper to avoid dehydration	Place these in refrigeration or cooler. If the cooling device is unavailable, place all insect material into the preservative	Place these in refrigeration or cooler. If the cooling device is unavailable, place all insect material into the preservative
	Hot water fix (larvae/full puparia)	Hot water is taken to the field via a thermos flask or available at the crime scene station set up by the agency overseeing the crime scene. Place larvae, pupae in hot water (1 min) before placing them in preservative. Full puparia pierced, then placed in hot water, then in preservative	Obtain hot water from external source: e.g., take away food outlet. If no available hot water, then place insects directly into the preservative (document preservative on label)	Obtain hot water from an external source: e.g., take away food outlet or place insects directly into preservative (document preservative on label)

Category	Specific Entomological Aspect	Gold Standard	Silver Standard	Bronze Standard
	Killing method (adults)	Spray a bottle of ethanol to spray directly onto the insect collected in the net then place in 70% alcohol	Dipping insects caught in the net into preservative and placed into 70% alcohol	Not applicable as adults; not collected
	Preservative (eggs/larvae /full and empty puparia) for minPMI	70–80% ethanol	Isopropyl alcohol, formalin or methanol (document preservative on label)	Any white-coloured alcohol (≥40% proof) obtained from a liquor outlet (document preservative on label)
Preservation of insects for toxicological analyses	Larvae, full and empty puparia	−20 °C	Freezer	Freezer
Preservation of insects for molecular analyses	Eggs, larvae, full and empty puparia, adults	100% ethanol	Freezer or if a preservative liquid is used (document preservative on label)	Freezer or if a preservative liquid is used (document preservative on label)
Transportation	Storage of insects for transporting	Refrigeration or cooler with frozen ice packs	If live insects are retained, then place them in a cooler with frozen ice packs	Not applicable all specimens preserved

Category	**Specific Entomological Aspect**	**Gold Standard**	**Silver Standard**	**Bronze Standard**
Preparation of insects for rearing	Types of containers used for rearing	Plastic containers with feeding and bedding medium	Plastic containers provided by the police/agency at the crime scene	Any sealable container; all specimens preserved
Identification	Method of identification	Morphological identification keys, molecular methods, hyperspectral and CT imaging, tomography, chemical methods	FE will conduct an identification	FE will conduct an identification
Age determination	Method of age determination	Larval instar, ADD method, isomegalen/isomorphen method, growth tables, crime scene resembling study within a growth chamber	FE will conduct age determination	FE will conduct age determination
Expert verification	The person involved in the verification	Conducted by an alternate FE	Conducted by an alternate FE	Conducted by an alternate FE
	Findings needed to be verified	Species and age of the specimen	Conducted by FE	Conducted by FE
Documenta	Crime scene	Insect data	Notebook	Notebook

Category	Specific Entomological Aspect	Gold Standard	Silver Standard	Bronze Standard
tion		collection form		
	Decomposition stage	Determination based on carcass characteristics, photos and videos at the crime scene and the mortuary. Previous experience and referring to existing publications	Send photographic and video evidence from the crime scene to an FE	Send photographic and video evidence from the crime scene to an FE

Crime Scene and Health Pathology Facility

The procedures outlined can be classified into two primary categories according to the site where specific entomological analyses occur: either at the crime scene/pathology facility or in the entomology laboratory. Typically, forensic entomologists or their surrogates gather insect evidence either directly at a crime scene or later at a health pathology facility where postmortem examinations are routinely conducted. The authorities responsible for the remains, such as the police, pathologists, and medical examiners/coroners, assign them to these facilities. Subsequently, a request is made if insect material is present, in order to determine the minimum postmortem interval (minPMI) and/or to provide a broad overview of the entomological circumstances at the crime scene [446].

At any of the aforementioned locations, a forensic entomologist (FE) or a designated representative must perform a series of standard tasks as outlined in Table 1. These tasks involve gathering essential data from the crime scene, either by physically being present or through the use of video and photographic documentation. This data includes environmental conditions, insect specimens, and various insect remnants such as mouth parts, appendages, wings, and empty puparia. Upon collection, certain insect samples may be preserved and stored, while others are placed on a growth medium for rearing purposes. Subsequently, both live and deceased specimens are transported to an entomology laboratory for in-depth analysis. It is imperative for the FE or proxy to strictly adhere to the general protocol established by the law enforcement agency overseeing the crime scene. Similar to all other investigative personnel present, the FE or proxy must don appropriate attire and utilize personal protective equipment like closed-toed shoes, long pants, scrubs, disposable overalls, and masks to minimize the risk of potential contamination and exposure to biohazards [446].

In order to effectively carry out their responsibilities, it is essential for field entomologists to visit locations with the appropriate tools and documentation to achieve three primary objectives. Firstly, they must gather insects, both live and deceased, using specially labeled plastic containers and vials, along with essential supplies such as a handheld lens, insulated bottle of hot water, forceps, fine-tipped artist paint brushes, an insect net, bedding materials like dry sand, sawdust, vermiculite, and food sources such as beef or pork pieces for rearing purposes. Ethanol, or ethyl alcohol, is also necessary for the killing and preservation of insects. Secondly, they should collect microclimatic data utilizing a portable weather gauge, an infrared thermometer, and a device for logging temperature data. Lastly, the entomologists need to record relevant information through prepared data entry sheets. Prior knowledge of the standard operating procedures of law enforcement at a specific location is vital for field entomologists to determine whether additional equipment such as a camera and video recorder is necessary for their tasks [446].

Collection of Onsite Data

The gathering and safeguarding of entomological evidence from a crime scene should be promptly conducted following the discovery of a body. Postponed documentation and sampling of insects could result in inaccurate data due to the ever-changing behaviour of carrion insects, influenced by weather changes, investigator actions, and scavenging by other animals [457, 458].

In order to mitigate the potential risks of damage and contamination, it is imperative for the law enforcement agency to adhere to specific protocols when preserving insect evidence at a crime scene. When establishing a perimeter around the crime scene, it is crucial for law enforcement to take into account the presence of insect activity in and around a deceased body, depending on the stage of decomposition and the age of the immature insects found on the body. While eggs and feeding larval stages of flies are typically limited to the body itself, post-feeding larval and pupal stages can be scattered beneath the body, in the surrounding soil near the body, or even buried at a certain distance from the body. When inside a dwelling, these stages may be discovered in close proximity to physical objects near the body, such as underneath carpets, inside cupboards, and among other household items [459].

Additionally, the movement of adult flies within residential buildings may be impacted by nearby attractions for flies, including lights, windows, and mirrors. It is ideal, when feasible, to visit an outdoor crime scene during daylight hours for entomological investigations. This allows for a better view of the surroundings of the crime scene and takes advantage of the fact that most insect activity occurs during the day. Unfortunately, the use of artificial lighting at night near a crime scene can draw in a variety of other unwanted insects, potentially disrupting the usual insect behaviour near the remains [450].

It is imperative to request all relevant information regarding the management of the crime scene from the lead forensic investigator. This includes obtaining photographs and videos taken during the initial visits to the scene by investigators, as well as any evidence of physical changes made to the immediate surroundings following the discovery of the remains (e.g., opening or closing windows, adjusting heating or cooling systems, and positioning light sources for nighttime investigations). One potential source of bias at a crime scene is providing the forensic entomologist (FE) or their representative with information about the last sighting of the deceased. Ideally, such details should only be disclosed after the minimum post-mortem interval has been determined by the FE [448].

Upon arriving at a crime scene and collaborating with law enforcement officials, the forensic entomologist or designated proxy should have the ability to inspect the remains and carefully observe the patterns of insects found on and around the carcass. Subsequent to this initial evaluation, the forensic entomologist or proxy can determine the necessary tools needed to effectively investigate the scene. In certain instances, there may be significant larval clusters present within and in close proximity to the natural openings of the carcass, such as the mouth, nostrils, ears, and genital area. These anatomical regions offer protection and contain suitable soft tissues for larval sustenance during the early phases of development. Additionally, these initial colonization sites can also manifest on other areas of the body depending on variables like surface moisture, thermal insulation, body positioning, attire, and the covering of wounds and bodies [460, 461].

When corpses are suspended above the ground, bodily fluids and insect larvae are expelled and fall onto the surface directly below the body, referred to as the 'drip zone'. Similarly, if corpses are contained within luggage, clusters of fly eggs might be evident on the visible zippers of the luggage. These findings regarding the initial stage of fly egg laying and larvae gathering can offer valuable clues for determining circumstances before death, including the cause and method of demise [461- 463].

The examination of carrion decay is an essential component of the fundamental education required to become a forensic entomologist, which commonly involves identifying the specific stage of decomposition of a human body. The patterns of insect colonization linked with various stages of decomposition can offer insights into estimating the minimum postmortem interval (minPMI). Typically, the process of body decomposition on land consists of five primary phases: freshly deceased, inflated, actively decaying, significantly decayed, and dried/remaining stages. Conversely, when in water, the decomposition process generally involves six stages: submersed freshly deceased, early buoyant, floating decay, inflated decay, floating remaining, and sunken remaining phases [458- 469].

When considering a preexisting stage of decomposition, it is important to calculate the expected time needed to reach this stage while taking into account various influencing factors. These factors directly impact the chemical makeup of the carcass and consequently influence insect colonization patterns. Factors such as climatic conditions (such as temperature, humidity, and photoperiod), accessibility for flies (including concealment and dwelling location), and the manner of death (such as hanging, burning, or drowning) all play a role in this process. In cases of hanging corpses, it is necessary to collect samples from both the body itself and the area directly beneath the body where decomposition fluids may have seeped into the soil. A minor burn on the body may actually attract insects due to the exposure of underlying tissues, while a more severe burn can deter insect activity. It is important to take into consideration the unique circumstances surrounding each case of cadaver decomposition in order to accurately assess the estimated time until a specific stage is reached. Climatic conditions, fly accessibility, and cause of death are all significant factors to consider when analyzing insect colonization patterns during decomposition [406].

When a dead body is placed in water, it diminishes the interest of land-dwelling animals while enhancing the likelihood of aquatic organisms being drawn to it. The size and age of the body play a role in determining the composition and quantity of flesh and bodily fluids, which in turn affect the colonization of insects and the process of decomposition. It is essential to take note of any additional sources in the vicinity that could potentially affect the attraction of insects to the body, such as garbage receptacles, restrooms, waste disposal areas, and other dead bodies. These factors can have a significant impact on the abundance of insects and the patterns of succession [423].

Collection of Microclimatic Data at a Crime Scene

Insects are ectothermic organisms, meaning their body temperatures vary with the temperatures of their surroundings to maintain internal stability. As such, when studying insects present at crime scenes, it is important to consider the ambient temperatures, as these can influence the growth and lifecycle patterns of carrion insects. More specifically, temperature plays a crucial role in the development, movement, metamorphosis, reproduction, and dormancy of insects. On the other hand, changes in temperature can also alter the succession patterns of insects as they impact the microbial processes involved in the decomposition of carcasses [467- 470].

The most reliable source for obtaining environmental temperature readings at a crime scene is by matching the temperature data from the nearest meteorological station with the conditions at the crime scene itself. Investigators have the option to request daily or hourly temperature information for the days leading up to the discovery of the remains. However, if the deceased is found inside a building, the meteorological station data will only be useful if there are openings such as windows, doors, and vents connecting the indoor and outdoor spaces. In these cases, the outdoor temperature data should be combined with the indoor temperatures when creating a thermal simulation model for the crime scene environment [472, 473].

In cases where the indoor environment is regulated using heating, cooling, and ventilation systems, the temperatures generated by these mechanisms should be included in the temperature data analysis. These temperatures should be compared to the actual temperature readings at the location. To accurately determine the hourly or minimum/maximum temperatures at a crime scene, a temperature data logging device can be utilized near the body and shielded with a

Stevenson screen. It is recommended to enhance the accuracy of meteorological data by performing a site-specific error calculation through regression analysis in order to estimate the minimum post-mortem interval (minPMI) [474, 475].

In addition to monitoring environmental temperatures, it is imperative to also document the temperatures of the body, water, soil, and larval mass in relation to the crime scene. A non-contact infrared thermometer can be utilized to measure the temperatures of the body and larval mass, while a temperature probe can be used to record the temperatures of the soil and water. The choice of which temperature data is most pertinent for estimating the minimum Post-Mortem Interval (minPMI) should be based on the level of heat transfer necessary for larval development. Specifically, the aggregated temperature of the larval mass (maggot mass) should be taken into consideration for minPMI calculations. Typically, large larval masses can be up to 20 °C higher than the surrounding temperature. Therefore, when identifying larvae as part of a larval mass, this heat source becomes crucial for the growth of late second-instar and third-instar larvae, rather than the ambient temperature [446].

It is crucial to document severe weather phenomena, such as intense rainfall during a specific time frame, as these occurrences could impact the migration, growth, and lifecycle sequences of scavenger insects. The levels of moisture and duration of daylight should also be documented in conjunction with temperature readings. The phase of the moon should not be overlooked, as a waxing gibbous moon could influence the movement of adult blowflies. This data is essential for replicating crime scene conditions or conducting a scientific study in a controlled environment to evaluate the growth rate of fly larvae [476, 477].

Recovery of Insects for Storage or Rearing Purposes

The evidence gathered at a crime scene should encompass a diverse range of insect development stages, including eggs, larvae, puparia, and adults, representing various insect groups such as flies, beetles, mites, and moths found on both the body and their immediate surroundings. Sufficient numbers of specimens at each developmental stage are necessary for conducting a variety of forensic entomology analyses in the lab, including species identification, estimation of post-mortem interval (PMI), and determination of foreign substances. The quantity of samples needed can vary depending on their availability, ranging from a single egg or larva to multiple egg clusters and groups of larvae [478].

At a crime scene, it is recommended to separate insects into two groups: one set for preservation and the other for raising until they reach the adult stage. Typically, this procedure is carried out on-site, however, if necessary, tools are lacking, the insects should be chilled (not frozen) to impede their growth and promptly sent to a laboratory. Preserved specimens are utilized for species identification, evaluation of their age by examining their instar stage, measuring larval length and width, as well as extracting gut contents for genetic and toxicological testing [479].

Preservation of Insects

Insects found on a body should be promptly preserved at the location of collection, as discussed earlier. If these insects are instead kept alive in containers without proper refrigeration for preservation at a later time, their age status may change, potentially leading to increased instances of cannibalistic behaviour and a decrease in the number of larvae available for future examination. In these situations, the development rate of the insects is compromised, rendering such samples unsuitable for estimating the minimum post-mortem interval (minPMI). [480]. If a comprehensive record of the thermal past of a specimen is provided, a forensic entomologist should possess the capability to deduce the age of insects at the time of collection and extract valuable details regarding the minimum postmortem interval for the investigators. Estimating the postmortem interval (PMI) for fly eggs and adult stages can prove challenging, given the limited information available for only a select few species. Nonetheless, in certain instances, these life stages constitute the sole samples obtained, and an experienced forensic entomologist might be able to discern the morphological alterations that take place during egg embryogenesis. Additionally, they can employ techniques outlined by Tyndale-Biscoe (1984) to determine the age of adult flies, particularly those found indoors. Subsequent to the discovery of eggs, they can be carefully collected after distinguishing them from soil and debris particles using a handheld magnifying glass and a fine-tipped artist's brush [481-483].

Alternatively, adult flies present at the location can be captured using an insect net. Once caught, they can easily be eliminated by immersing or spraying them with 70% alcohol before transferring the deceased specimen to a vial. If alcohol is not accessible, the adult fly can be caught in the net and placed cautiously into an insect-killing jar for preservation. Another option is to utilize insect sticky paper during the day to attract and gather adult flies effortlessly. After gathering them, individual flies can be taken out from the sticky paper using a precise paintbrush and vegetable oil [484].

When gathering fragile young first and second-instar larvae, it is recommended to use a delicate paintbrush with a fine tip. As for older pre- and post-third instar larvae and those in the pupal stage, they can be extracted using forceps or a specially designed spoon that fits into a collection vial. Unlike forceps, which are only suitable for individual larva collection, a spoon is capable of gathering a substantial number of larvae from a surface or larval aggregation. These collected larvae should then be immersed in hot water (not boiling) for about a minute before being transferred into vials containing 80% ethanol. To ensure the preservation of the morphological characteristics of the insect undergoing metamorphosis, it is advisable to puncture fully formed puparia with a pin prior to immersion in hot water and subsequent submersion in 70–80% ethanol [485- 487].

The necessary hot water can be transported to the location in a thermos flask or insulated bottle, and may also be available at a nearby café or take-away establishment. It is essential to affix a suitable label on the outer surface of the vials before storing them, using indelible ink to specify the time, date, sampling location, collector's name, and body part from which the sample was taken. Additionally, a duplicate label containing the same details should be placed inside the vial using a pencil as it will not dissolve in alcohol [399].

Beetles found at the scene of a crime should be carefully selected using forceps and hot water, and then immersed in 70% ethanol to ensure their preservation. To observe beetles more closely, one can conduct a detailed examination of the debris near the body and sift through the soil beneath the body up to a depth of about 20 centimeters. It is important to note that individuals with lower-ranking titles should gather all insects found in connection with the deceased and defer to a forensic entomologist for further analysis [488].

When faced with a crime scene situated in a water-based environment, it is advisable to gather the larval phases of freshwater insects like mayflies, stone flies, and caddis flies using forceps and place them in plastic vials filled with 70% ethanol. Furthermore, it is advisable for Silver and Bronze level personnel to collect all aquatic fauna found in connection with the deceased. Conversely, it is suggested to preserve around 40% of sampled specimens from remains found at the bottom of streams in appropriately labeled vials with 95% ethanol to prevent decay while in storage [489].

The live aquatic insects retrieved from a cadaver should be transferred to a laboratory for further study and categorization. These insects should be accommodated in plastic containers filled with water sourced from their original habitat, such as a lake, sea, pond, or stream. While in transit, it is recommended to keep the specimens cool by placing the container on ice, with periodic ventilation by intermittently opening the lid [466].

Preparation of Insects at the Crime Scene for Rearing Purposes

Live insects gathered from the crime scene for breeding purposes should be placed on a dish, such as a Petri dish or foil, along with an appropriate food source, such as meat. This dish should then be positioned on a layer of bedding material, such as sawdust, vermiculite, or builders' sand, within a container equipped with a mesh lid. When preparing fully developed puparia for transport to the laboratory, they can be transferred directly into containers that are half-filled with bedding material and sealed with a standard lid. No additional food source or ventilation is necessary if all insect specimens are transported in a cooler or refrigerated environment [406].

Laboratory

The subsequent sections address the responsibilities of a Forensic Entomologist in examining either the specimens they have collected themselves or those collected by a proxy. These duties involve the identification and measurement of larval, pupal, and adult external characteristics, as well as the rearing of immature specimens to the adult stage. An entomology laboratory should be equipped with essential tools such as stereo microscopes, vernier calipers, growth chambers or temperature-controlled environments, preservative chemicals like ethanol, protective gloves, forceps, scalpels, and Petri dishes. Additional equipment like DNA/RNA reagent kits, PCR machines, and genetic sequencers may also be necessary for insect identification. It is important to handle carrion insects, whether alive or deceased, with caution when bringing them into the laboratory to facilitate a range of analyses [490].

Identification

The initial step in the analysis should involve identifying the specimens to the species level. This is crucial as without this information, the accuracy of subsequent analyses may be compromised. Typically, insect identifications rely on either morphological or molecular methods. While alternative techniques like hyperspectral or CT imaging, tomography, and chemical methods can also be employed, each method has its own set of advantages and disadvantages depending on cost and accessibility. Nonetheless, regardless of the approach taken, the objective should be to achieve the most accurate identification possible. Ideally, the most comprehensive and precise identification can be obtained by sending the collected specimens pertaining to the minimum postmortem interval (minPMI) to a dipteran taxonomist. The following sections will delve into the two primary methods utilized for insect identification: morphological identification and molecular identification [491- 493].

Identification of carrion insects at the species level through morphological analysis can be achieved by utilizing taxonomic keys along with standard or electron microscopic images. These dichotomous keys offer a systematic approach by assessing morphological characteristics that assist in species identification. Proficiency in entomology and extensive experience is essential for utilizing taxonomic keys effectively and accurately for species determination, especially through microscopic examination to differentiate various morphological traits of specimens. There are numerous comprehensive keys available for identifying flies, including proposed keys focusing on specific species, developmental stages, and geographic locations. On the other hand, taxonomic keys for forensically important beetles are less abundant by comparison [494- 505].

Ultrastructural analysis using scanning electron microscopes (SEM) plays a crucial role in accurately identifying different fly species at various stages of their life cycle, including eggs, larvae, puparia, and adults. Key ultrastructural features observed in eggs include the micropylar plate, median area, respiratory plastron, hatching lines, and chorion sculpturing. Larval characteristics that aid in species identification include posterior spiracles, respiratory slits, peritreme ornamentation, anterior spiracles, cephaloskeleton, and spine arrangement. For full puparia, distinguishing features such as bubble membranes, respiratory horns, spine arrangements, and posterior spiracles are closely examined and related to their larval structures. Distinctive characteristics of adult stages, including thoracic setae patterns and wing venation, are essential for species differentiation. Furthermore, SEM-based ultrastructural studies have also been conducted on forensically significant coleopteran species from families like Nitidulide and Carabidae. These studies focus on ultrastructural features such as antennomeres, head capsulae, and mouthparts [506- 511].

The use of molecular techniques, such as DNA barcoding, can be considered as an alternative for identifying insects associated with crime in cases where the user lacks taxonomic expertise but possesses the required laboratory skills. It may also be feasible to outsource the molecular analysis to a specialized laboratory. Furthermore, in instances where only a limited number of specimens or fragments lacking distinguishing features are available and there are no taxonomic keys to consult for the developmental stage of the collected samples, molecular methods offer a reliable approach to species identification [512- 514].

Deoxyribonucleic Acid (DNA) barcoding for insect identification aims to identify distinct short sequences of nucleotides within the genome of each species in order to differentiate them from closely related species. The use of Cytochrome

C oxidase subunit 1 (CO1), the final enzyme in the mitochondrial respiratory chain, is widely acknowledged as an effective marker for DNA barcoding in insects thanks to its stable mutation rate and consistent characteristics among different species [515, 516].

Typically, the process of identifying crime-collected specimens at a molecular level involves five key steps: sample preparation, DNA extraction, PCR amplification, sequencing, and sequence library identification. Specimens of adult, larval, and pupal flies preserved in 70% ethanol are suitable for DNA extraction. The primers necessary for PCR amplification can be acquired by consulting relevant literature. However, the lack of comprehensive genetic research on forensic flies in various global regions has resulted in a shortage of sequence data for these species in those areas [515].

Previous research studies have contributed DNA sequences for carrion flies, with Stevens and Wall (2001) providing data for *Calliphorid* species in the United Kingdom, Wallman *et al.* (2005) for *Calliphorid* species in Australia, Harvey *et al.* (2003) for specific species like *Calliphora dubia*, *Chrysomya rufifacies*, and *Lucilia cuprina*, Harvey *et al.* (2003) for Calliphorid species in Southern Africa and Australia, and a comprehensive global study on *Calliphorid* species conducted by Harvey *et al.* (2008)[516- 521].

Examining Larvae and Full Puparia for Age Determination

Developmental studies provide a framework for determining the age of immature flies, which can be valuable in estimating the minimum Post post-mortem interval (minPMI). The stage of fly larvae can be identified through a detailed examination of the number of respiratory openings present at their hind spiracles under a microscope. In general, first-stage blowfly larvae exhibit a single opening, while second and third-stage larvae display two and three openings, respectively. On the other hand, distinguishing between pre- and post-feeding phases of third-stage larvae involves observing changes in body colour (from translucent to opaque), a distended crop due to feeding, body compression, and a tendency to move away from the carcass [497].

Moreover, the dimensions of larvae can serve as an indicator of their age. These dimensions can be accurately assessed using a stage micrometer and a vernier caliper. Comparing the actual measurements of a sampled larva with established reference values from previous studies can help in estimating the age of the specimen, including the post-mortem interval (PMI). However, factors such as temperature fluctuations, food sources, and exposure to foreign substances can impact the accuracy of age determination. Magni *et al.* (2012) [514] utilized the length of dehydrated larvae of *Lucilia illustris* (Meigen) alongside dried larval specimens collected at a crime scene to determine their age. Various studies have provided reference values for changes in length for species like *Ch. megacephala* [523- 525], *Ch. rufifacies* [526, 527], *Ch. bezziana* [528], *L. sericata* [529], and *L. cuprina* [530].

Moreover, prior research has shown variations in the length and instar stage of larvae at different constant temperature conditions through the use of isomegalen and isomorphen curves. These curves have been utilized for species including *Calliphora vicina* (Robineae-Desvoidy), *L. sericata*, *Ch. albiceps*, *Protophormia terraenovae* (Robineae-Desvoidy), *Ch. megacephala*, and *Liopygia argyrostoma* (Robineae-Desvoidy) [529, 530].

Pupal morphogenesis is a significant factor to consider when estimating minPMI, as the intact puparia remain in proximity to carcasses for an extended period of time. The development of external organs in pupae can be analyzed by using a stereo microscope to inspect the puparium after its removal with precise instruments. A visual record of the external organ development in a selected pupa can be compared with a series of reference photographs from a previous publication to determine its age accurately. It is crucial to account for any variations in temperature that the intact puparia may have experienced prior to collection, as colder temperatures have the potential to delay the process of pupal morphogenesis [527].

Photographic timelines depicting the developmental stages of external organs in pupae during intra-puparium development have been provided for various insect species including *Megaselia spiracularis*, *Megaselia scalaris*, *Calliphora vicina*, *Hermetia illucens*, *Ch. Megacephala*, *Ch. rufifacies*, and *Dohrniphora cornuta* [528].

Laboratory-based techniques utilizing hyperspectral or CT imaging, tomography, as well as biomolecular and chemical methods, can be applied for the ageing of insect larvae and full puparia. These sophisticated techniques necessitate specialized instrumentation and a high level of expertise for accurate analysis [528-540].

Rearing

The process of nurturing eggs, larvae, and pupae until they reach adulthood can greatly assist in accurately identifying the species. Identifying species at the adult stage is more reliable, as they are thoroughly documented in taxonomic guides. When raising dipteran species in a controlled environment, it is essential to house them in insect cages and supply them with ample food, water, and suitable sites for egg-laying [541, 542].

Immature life stages are most effectively cultivated in controlled growth chambers where factors such as temperature, humidity, and photoperiod can be meticulously regulated. These studies of development are crucial in determining the time required to reach different developmental stages, as well as monitoring changes in larval size and shape. It is advised to use swine muscle as a larval food source in these growth chamber experiments, as the domestic pig (Sus scrofa L.) is commonly used as a surrogate for humans in developmental research. Furthermore, in cases involving wildlife-related crimes, the same type of tissue should be used as the feeding substrate in growth chamber experiments [543, 544].

Xenobiotic Detection

The use of insects in the detection of xenobiotics hinges on the extended retention of drugs, pesticides, and metals in their tissues, resulting in enhanced sensitivity for analytical detection methods [543].

At a crime scene, fly larvae in various stages of development - from larval to pupal to adult - can serve as a valuable source for the extraction and identification of chemicals. Research has demonstrated that larvae taken from internal organs like the liver, as well as from the head and muscles of a cadaver, retain significant concentrations of chemicals [544].

Larvae collected from these specific areas should be kept alive and deprived of food for several hours before analysis to promote the absorption of any chemicals into their metabolic systems. It is recommended that deceased larvae be stored in dry conditions at a temperature of -20 °C to maintain a high level of chemical retention and concentration, as storing them in ethanol may result in the loss of trace amounts of drugs [545, 546].

In the laboratory, various techniques can be utilized to prepare sampled fly development stages for analysis. These methods include maceration and homogenization, digestion using a potent acid or enzyme, and pulverization through grinding. The detection of xenobiotics in these samples can be achieved using analytical methods such as immunoassay, high-performance liquid chromatography (HPLC), liquid chromatography-mass spectrometry (LC-MS), and gas chromatography-mass spectrometry (GC-MS) [427].

Documentation

Documenting a crime scene is essential in order to protect the integrity of evidence and maintain the chain of custody without interruption. Research has indicated that the design of protocol sheets utilized by a forensic examiner may vary based on the specific needs and regulations of investigative agencies and legal frameworks in a particular geographic area. This documentation is comprised of two primary components: the procedures conducted at the crime scene, which involve information collected by either the forensic examiner or a designated proxy, and the subsequent laboratory procedures, which entail information exclusively handled by the forensic examiner. Following the completion of these procedures, the forensic examiner should possess adequate information to formulate an articulate expert witness statement (Table 2) [547-550].

Table 2: Specific information that needs to be included in protocol sheets. Many review papers also list such protocols and should be consulted [398]

Type of Protocol	Category	Specific Information
Crime scene/autopsy	General case information	Date, case number, date and time of scene examination, name of the FE and investigation officer(s)
	Prior information from investigation officer (**IMPORTANT**)	Location found date and time body recovered. The date when reported missing of the decedent and date and time last seen alive **SHOULD** only be available following the calculated minPMI to avoid bias in the analyses
	Recordings of the body	Position of body's main axis, the position of extremities, and position of head and face, the location of the body in reference to vegetation, and proximity to open doors, windows, or other openings if within a structure, description of clothing, type of debris on the body, level exposure of the body (open air or burial; full sun or shade exposure), any detectable alterations to the body (i.e., natural, man-made, and scavenging marks)
	Recordings of the crime location (outdoor)	General habitat (rural or urban, terrestrial, or aquatic), sun or shade conditions, type of terrestrial ecosystem (1. rural; forest, tillable land, pasture, and crop, 2. urban; vacant lot, pavement, and rubbish container), type of aquatic ecosystem (lake, river, pond, irrigation canal, swamp, marshland), aquatic water type (fresh, brackish, and saltwater)

Type of Protocol	Category	Specific Information
	Recordings of the crime location (Indoor)	Type of building (open or closed), doors and windows closed or open, on or off fans, lights, A/C and heaters
	Recordings of insect activity	Location of insect aggregations on the body, location of dispersing larvae, full and empty puparia up to 10 m away from the body. Attention should be given to the presence of ants
	Recordings at autopsy	Date and time of body placed into refrigeration after coming from the scene and removed prior to autopsy, locations of specimens (in/on the body, clothing and other covers, body bag)
	Climate data (temperature)	Ambient temperature, larval mass temperature, temperature readings of A/C and heaters, moon phases
	Attachments	Diagram of the body showing locations of insect mass infestations and sample locations, weather data from the nearest meteorological station, photos of body in situ, autopsy photographs
Laboratory	Insect sampling	Sampled numbers (live and dead), type of insect (flies, beetles, or mites), growth stages (eggs, larvae, full and empty puparia, and adults)
	Sampling method	Fixation and preservation medium (% alcohol), date and time of preservation and fixation, sampled location (water, soil or arial)
	Identification	Identification method (morphological or

Type of Protocol	Category	Specific Information
		molecular), specific species identified
	Age determination	Method of age determination, minPMI estimation based on available data

Typically, a Forensic Entomologist (FE) will conduct a single visit to a crime scene, highlighting the importance of thorough documentation during this initial visit. In some cases, a return visit may be necessary to gather additional contextual information and collect more insect samples, especially if the initial visit took place at night. To streamline the sampling process without compromising detailed record-keeping, it is advisable to utilize a protocol sheet featuring specific questions with multiple-choice options to capture crucial details about the crime scene, including crime characteristics, microclimatic data, quantity and quality of specimens collected, and information about the individual conducting the sampling. Furthermore, a laboratory data sheet should be prepared to meticulously record all laboratory analyses performed, serving as a reference for verification by experts [406].

Referring to the Literature

The ability to accurately determine a successful entomological analysis of a crime scene relies heavily on the practical experience gained by a forensic entomologist over the course of their profession. One of the most effective methods for acquiring and enhancing the expertise and abilities related to insects in forensic investigations is by consulting previously published studies and casework. These resources serve as valuable references for practitioners in integrating existing knowledge into protocols, as well as offering a thorough framework for scholars and researchers to establish training programs and engage in further investigations [550].

Fly Development Studies

Studies on developmental patterns provide insights into the variations in the life history of flies. The information obtained from these studies can be utilized directly to calculate the minimum post-mortem interval (minPMI), as they typically include detailed life history tables and curves depicting developmental stages. By analyzing the timeline data and lower temperature thresholds for development provided in these tables, one can determine the accumulated degree-days/hours (ADD/ADH) required for development, therefore estimating the minPMI. However, when selecting a previous developmental study to support an estimation of minPMI for a specific fly species, it is crucial to consider factors such as temperature conditions, photoperiod, humidity levels, larval diet, and the geographic origin of the source populations to ensure accuracy [551, 552]. These studies not only offer the foundational information necessary for determining minimum post-mortem interval (minPMI), but also emphasize the importance of adhering to stringent laboratory protocols when carrying out experiments pertaining to crime scenes. The protocols should outline procedures for generating and maintaining colonies, ensuring genetic diversity, simulating environmental conditions in an insectary or growth chamber, and collecting larval samples and data. Several researchers have undertaken developmental investigations on various species of blow flies (Table 3) [552].

Table 3. Development studies were conducted on some forensically important fly species from different global regions. This table presents an overview only and is a starting point for any person interested in forensic entomology

Species	Reference Studies with Study Locations
Ch. megacephala, *Ch. rufifacies*, *Ch. albiceps*, *L. sericata*, *L. cuprina*, *L. illustris*, *Calliphora vomitoria* (L.), *C. vicina*, *Phormia regina* (Meigen)	Bambaradeniya *et al.* (2023) (Asia, middle east, Australia, Europe) [420], Niederegger *et al.* (2010) (Germany) [553], Wang *et al.* (2016) (China) [554], Greenberg and Tantawi (1993) (USA) [555], Ames and Turner (2003) (UK) [556], Ireland and Turner (2006) (UK) [557], Niederegger *et al.* (2013) (Germany) [558], Wood *et al.* (2022) (UK) [559], Donovan *et al.* (2006) (UK) [560], Hwang and Turner (2009) (UK) [561], Aak *et al.* (2011) (Norway) [562], Sanei- Dehkordi *et al.* (2014) (Iran) [563], Baque *et al.* (2015) (Germany) [564], Byrd and Allen (2001) (USA) [565], Nabity *et al.* (2007) (USA) [566], Roe (2014) (USA) [567], Roe and Higley (2023) (USA) [568]
Sarcophaga rufucornis (Fabricius)	Sukhapanth *et al.* (1988) (Thailand) [569], Amoudi *et al.* (1994) (Saudi Arabia) [570], Nassu *et al.* (2014) (Brazil) [571], Adhikari *et al.* (2016) (India) [572], Bansode *et al.* (2016) (India) [573], Barbosa *et al.* (Brazil) [574]
M. scalaris	Prawirodisastro and Benjamin (1979) (USA) [575], Trumble and Pienkowski (1979) (USA) [576], Greenberg and Wells (1998) (USA) [577], Harrison and Cooper (2003) (USA) [578], Zuha *et al.* (2012) (Malaysia) [579], Feng and Liu (2014) (China) [533], Zuah and Omar (2014)

Species	Reference Studies with Study Locations
	(Malaysia) [580], Chakraborty *et al.* (2016) (India) [581], Thomas *et al.* (2016) (USA) [185], Ong *et al.* (2018) (Malaysia) [582], Castillo-Alanis *et al.* (2020) (Mexico) [583]

Insect Successional Studies

Insect successional research elucidates the process of insect colonization in decomposing carcasses. These investigations can be either observational or experimental, with the primary goal of collecting data on insect species present, environmental conditions, and characteristics of decomposition stages [585].

Observational-based successional studies are typically carried out to illustrate seasonal and ecosystem transformations in both terrestrial and aquatic environments, while experimental studies examine various death and carcass scenarios. Data obtained from successional studies can be used to assist in understanding insect ecology and behaviour at crime scenes, especially when considering the geographic location and temperature correlations. Matuszewski *et al.* (2019) [585] provided a comprehensive overview of global successional studies involving different carcass types in a variety of ecosystems [585, 586].

Casework

From time to time, a report emerges that presents a blend of factual information and expert analysis by a forensic entomologist who has analyzed a specific crime scene. This report can offer valuable insights for the current investigation, guiding the creation of a thorough witness statement and suggesting areas that could benefit from additional research. Kotzé *et al.* (2021) [587] have outlined 16 subheadings that may be pertinent in compiling a forensic entomology report, highlighting the importance of staying current with the latest methodologies [587].

Identification of Diptera Puparia in Forensic and Archeo-Funerary Contexts

In the field of forensics, insects and other environmental organisms, such as microbes, algae, and plants, can offer valuable insights to address investigative inquiries, which are commonly referred to as the 6Ws in English (When, Where, What, How, Who, and Why). Forensic entomology specifically involves the utilization of information about insects and arthropods in legal contexts, and it has been evolving since the late 19th century primarily to determine the minimum post-mortem interval (min PMI), or more precisely the time since death [588-590].

Furthermore, advancements in the understanding of insect phenology, habitats, and distribution over the past century have led to the utilization of insects in addressing a broader range of inquiries. These inquiries include determining the time of death, identifying the primary crime scene, detecting drugs, and even conducting DNA identification of victims when the body is absent but insect larvae or puparia are still present at the scene. This methodology has proven effective with the analysis of beetle frass as well [591- 594].

Funerary archeoentomology is closely related to the study of insect colonization on human and animal remains, sharing common techniques and expertise with forensic entomology. Despite these similarities, the two fields are distinct and separate disciplines [593].

Forensic entomology is based on four important principles:

1. Insect development is influenced by temperature, species characteristics, and population dynamics. This knowledge allows for the estimation of minimum post-mortem intervals (minPMI) over short time periods when the temperature history of initial colonizers is known [595, 596].

2. The sequence in which insects infest a cadaver follows certain patterns and can be somewhat anticipated. This enables the calculation of minimum Post-Mortem Interval (minPMI) over extended periods based on the entomological community found on the body or remains.

3. Different species exhibit distinct habitat preferences and life cycles, allowing for the determination of the time of death in older cases and the assessment of post-mortem body relocation. It has been emphasized that the landscape structure must also be taken into account as it significantly influences species distribution. Furthermore, climate change is having a notable impact on the phenology and distribution of species, resulting in prolonged activity during cooler seasons or displaying bimodal life cycles. The introduction of new species to faraway regions is leading to a more uniform global carrion entomofauna, especially among crucial forensic indicators such as blowflies, house flies, and flesh flies [597- 600].

4. The impact of pharmaceutical substances on the growth and maturation of insects is species-specific, with certain species experiencing either a boost or a hindrance in development rate, while others remain largely unaffected. This finding underscores the necessity of comprehensive understanding regarding the ramifications of various types of drugs on various species [591].

It is clear from these arguments that the commencement of any entomological inquiry, whether in the realm of forensic science or within other disciplines like medicine, agriculture, archaeology, etc., necessitates the accurate identification of the species and their life stages. This fundamental requirement can be met through the comparative analysis of specimens with the typus preserved in a public collection, as outlined in the International Code of Zoological Nomenclature, a key principle familiar to entomologists and zoologists [601].

The process is typically effective when examining adult specimens, as species descriptions are primarily based on mature specimens. However, a practical approach involves utilizing dichotomous identification keys for specimen identification. This method is particularly efficient when focusing on adult specimens. In forensic entomology, the majority of samples collected by crime scene investigators or during autopsies consist of immature stages such as larvae, puparia, or remnants of their presence in older cases or archeo-funerary contexts. It is important to note that the number of fly larvae may vary during the colonization process, while the number of puparia generally increases until the last larva has undergone pupation. The gradual decline in the number of puparia over time is influenced by predation, dispersion, and taphonomic processes (Figure 34) [601].

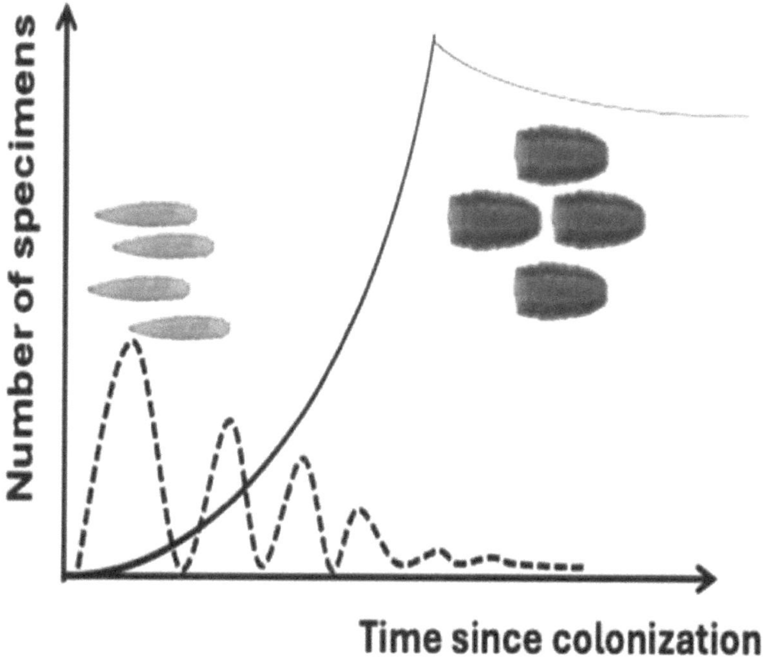

Figure 34: A diagram illustrating the pattern of larvae (represented by a dashed line) and puparia (represented by a solid line) over the period of colonization. The gradual decline in puparia numbers over time can be attributed to factors such as predation, dispersal, and taphonomic processes.[601]

In recent times, there have been advancements in the development of identification keys for certain larvae. In Europe, it is relatively easy to identify most larvae of the Calliphoridae family, as well as some genera of the Fanniidae and Muscidae families that are of interest in forensic studies. However, there is a noticeable disparity when it comes to identifying puparia. Despite some older sources, scattered descriptions in general literature, and only a few recent publications, there remains a significant gap in understanding the puparia of many species relevant to forensic investigations. Furthermore, there is a lack of research on the puparia of other families [602- 612].

When morphological traits are difficult to observe or unavailable, the most frequently utilized method for identification is molecular, relying on the analysis of DNA. Additionally, in recent times, chemical analysis of cuticles has demonstrated encouraging outcomes, although it does not encompass all species of forensic significance at present. Although several methods have been proposed for identifying puparium, there is a conspicuous absence of organized and clearly defined strategies. Therefore, the objective of this paper is to comprehensively outline the frequently employed techniques for puparium identification [613-615].

Definition, Structure, and Formation of Puparia

In 2016, Martin-Vega and colleagues provided a comprehensive and accurate explanation of the pupariation process along with a revision in the naming conventions. Within cyclorrhaphous flies, the pupal stage and the following growth of the pharate adult take place within a solid, barrel-shaped puparium made from the third instar larva's cuticle. This stage, lasting from the formation of the puparium to the emergence of the adult, makes up over half of the overall immature development, and once the puparium is formed, it does not show any external signs of ageing [616].

Moreover, the recovery of puparia from a body or a crime scene serves as the sole direct evidence of a species' presence following adult emergence and dispersal. The chemical stability of chitin allows puparia to potentially endure for centuries or even millennia. The state of the puparium, whether closed (representing the prepupa, pupa, and pharate adult stages) or open after adult emergence, depends on the different developmental phases taking place inside. It is common for some literature in the forensic entomology field to incorrectly use the term "pupa" when referring to the closed puparium. However, it is important to avoid using the term "pupa" as it specifically pertains to a particular developmental stage occurring within the puparium for a limited duration, without acknowledging the prepupa and pharate adult stages [617, 618].

Morphology-Based Approach

The field of morphology is a long-standing, conventional, and direct method of recognition. This process entails examining distinct anatomical characteristics of interest and cross-referencing them with established morphological descriptions or utilizing identification aids. In the realm of forensic Diptera, existing research predominantly concentrates on specific fly groups (such as Calliphoridae, Muscidae, and Piophilidae) which offer comprehensive information for mature specimens. Nevertheless, descriptions of immature stages are often limited. Challenges primarily stem from the scarcity of distinguishing traits exhibited by eggs, larvae, and puparia (as depicted in Figure 35), along with the variability in the usefulness of these features for species differentiation [611].

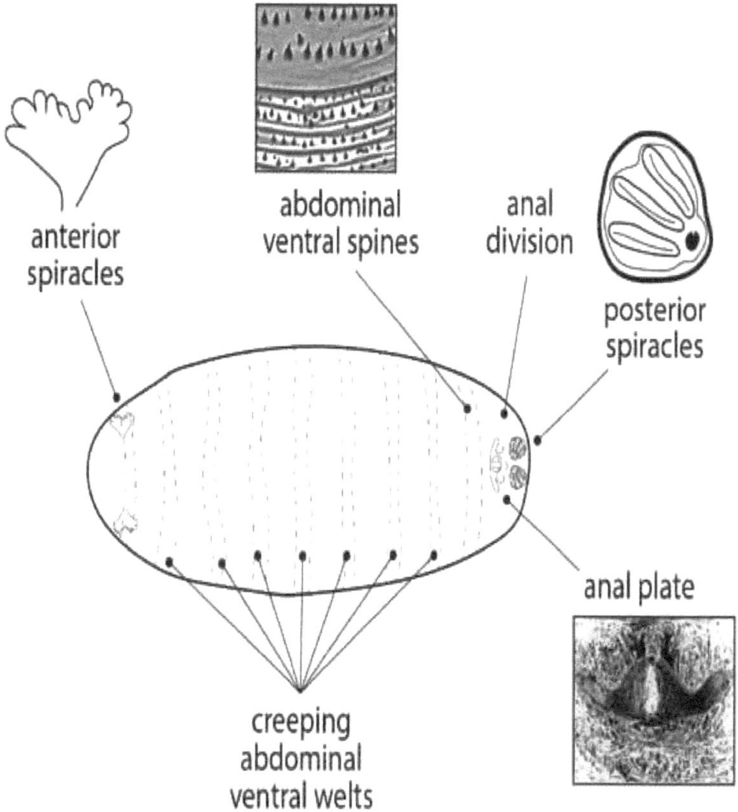

Figure 35: The diagnostic features of Diptera puparia are examined through ventral views and anatomical details. Schematic representations are used to analyze puparia for species identification. While each element is accurately portrayed from photographs, the overall depiction is not realistic due to the lack of scale and elements being selected from various species [611].

Furthermore, puparia commonly exhibit similarities to the larval stage, but physical changes such as contraction during pupariation can lead to a partial reduction in detail. Moreover, oral sclerites may not always be evident in the empty puparia, particularly in older cases and within archaeological settings where puparia are a prevalent discovery among Diptera specimens. Consequently, adult fragments are rare and typically poorly preserved in such scenarios, with a significant loss in distinguishing features like setae, portions of leg segments, antennae, and palpi [617- 620].

In certain cases and within specific families, the absence of the anterior part of the puparium post-adult emergence, coupled with the preservation of oral sclerites, presents challenges in identifying species at a detailed level, potentially rendering it extremely challenging, if not entirely unattainable. It is important to recognize that while certain features may serve as useful diagnostic markers for specific taxa, they may not offer the same level of relevance for others. For instance, within the realm of forensic investigations, the presence of posterior spiracles holds significance in blow flies (Calliphoridae) and Hydrotaea Robineau-Desvoidy, 1830 house flies (Muscidae), yet provides limited insight in Piophilidae, wherein anterior spiracles play a more crucial role, particularly when identifying genus distinctions [621].

The proposal of breeding specimens has been suggested as a resolution to address the difficulty of identifying puparia. This strategy proves successful only if the organisms housed within the puparia remain alive, are carefully gathered, and are transported to the entomological laboratory without compromising their viability. Regrettably, this method is not applicable in cases where empty puparia are encountered or when attempts to rear the immature organisms in the laboratory are unsuccessful. In such instances, it becomes essential to compare insect remnants to specimens housed in private or natural history museum collections and to work alongside taxonomic experts in order to accurately determine the species in question. An alternative approach involving DNA analysis may also be considered [621- 624].

Global warming and globalization have contributed to shifts in species distribution, with several non-native species of forensic importance now appearing in new areas. For instance, *Chrysomya megacephala* (Fabricius, 1794) has been observed in Portugal, Spain, and Malta in Europe, while *Synthesyomya nudiseta* Van Der Wulp, 1883 has been documented in Italy on human remains. The successful identification of a newly introduced species necessitates a comprehensive understanding that extends beyond just the local insect population. It also requires access to broad identification resources at the family or genus level rather than solely focusing on species found within a specific region. This underscores the importance of cultivating expert taxonomists with a deep understanding of various taxa, rather than just limited knowledge of local fauna or specific geographic regions. Regrettably, current research funding does not seem to prioritize these crucial aspects [625-628].

In the European context, the issue of a shortage of taxonomists has been extensively documented in the European Red List of Insect Taxonomists. Through a quantitative analysis of taxonomic publications in scientific journals spanning the past decade, as well as an online survey, this red list offers an assessment of the taxonomic capabilities within each insect order and European Union country. It reveals that the taxonomic capacity is under threat or diminishing for 41.4% of insect orders at the European level. The four major insect orders (Coleoptera, Diptera, Lepidoptera, and Hymenoptera), which encompass insects of forensic significance, are addressed by over 80% of countries (with rates exceeding 90% for Coleoptera and Lepidoptera). Yet, the capacity to properly identify, describe, and name new insect species is only present in 26% (Coleoptera) to 58% (Hymenoptera) of all countries. Regrettably, Diptera are identified as having inadequate capacity at the European level. Although there is a lack of official studies, it appears that the state of European taxonomists is comparable, if not more dire, on other continents according to the knowledge of the authors [629].

Universities, museums, and institutes specializing in forensic entomology bear a considerable burden in tackling this matter. It is imperative to provide them with support on an international, national, and local scale to enhance their ability to identify species, particularly in the key groups relevant to forensic investigations. This assistance should not solely focus on the six primary families of flies (Calliphoridae, Sarcophagidae, Muscidae, Fanniidae, Phoridae, and Piophilidae) or beetles, but should also encompass specialized knowledge sharing, education, training, and opportunities for professional taxonomists. Furthermore, both local and global authorities must acknowledge the importance of allocating sufficient resources to sustain taxonomic expertise, which in certain instances may lead to the identification and prevention of public health concerns in both human and veterinary healthcare, such as instances of vector-borne diseases responsible for over 17% of all infectious diseases and more than 700,000 deaths annually [612].

DNA-Based Approach

Molecular identification is now commonly employed to complement conventional morphological examinations in validating species identification. Insects have the potential to be definitively identified through the sequencing of a unique DNA segment referred to as the “barcode”. The mitochondrial COI gene has been designated as the molecular focal point for discriminating multiple metazoan species due to its high inter-specific divergence and low intra-specific divergence, which denotes the rate of mutations between two DNA sequences [630- 632].

Mitochondrial targets, which are abundant in cells, exhibit a higher mutation rate compared to nuclear targets. The COI gene, spanning 1535 base pairs, codes for subunit I of Cytochrome Oxidase, a critical protein involved in the electron-transport chain of cellular respiration. Specifically, the 658 base pairs at the 5′ end of the gene are identified as the “barcoding region” and can be amplified using “universal primers”. Novel sets of primers designed to anneal within or between the barcoding region have been recently introduced. Although shorter barcode sequences have been successful in identifying *Fanniidae* species of forensic importance, it is advised not to utilize DNA fragments shorter than ~200 base pairs for distinguishing Sarcophagidae species [633- 637].

Utilizing multiple primer pairs, a technique known as "mini barcoding", enables the amplification of overlapping fragments that can be aligned using computational analysis, resulting in a longer nucleotide sequence. This method proves beneficial in enhancing amplification success in situations where DNA degradation is substantial or when dealing with ancient samples [635].

When closely related species display minimal inter-specific divergence, the analysis of the COI gene may not offer reliable discrimination, as evidenced in the case of *Lucilia caesar* (Linnaeus, 1758) and *Lucilia illustris* Meigen, 1826 (Diptera: Calliphoridae). In such scenarios, alternative genetic markers such as mitochondrial targets like COII, Cytb, ND5, and 28S rDNA, or nuclear targets like EF-1a, ITS1, ITS2, and PER can be employed. Furthermore, the combined use of these markers, referred to as "concatenation", presents an additional approach to enhance species resolution among closely related organisms. Nonetheless, recent advancements in whole genome sequencing have emerged as the most effective method in distinguishing congeneric species, particularly within the genus *Lucilia Robineau-Desvoidy*, 1830 [638- 647].

The primary benefit of utilizing genotyping for purposes of identification lies in its ability to be applied to any specimens, regardless of their developmental stages. This method has been proven effective for both adult and larval stages across all instars, although further exploration is necessary for its consistent application to puparia. This limitation is connected to the amount of accessible DNA, as the epithelial tissue (larval exuviae) that separates the metamorphosing fly from the puparium until the process is complete acts as the sole available source of DNA. In 2010, Mazzanti and his colleagues detailed the successful identification of 42 Diptera puparia recovered from crime scenes, with the oldest specimen being 20 years old at the time of DNA extraction [615].

Although the procedures for identifying insect species in laboratories are well-established, there are numerous pitfalls associated with interpreting data, which is a fundamental aspect of every scientific inquiry. Researchers worldwide create nucleotide sequences that populate reference DNA repositories like GenBank at the National Center for Biotechnology Information (NCBI) and the

European Bioinformatics Institute (EBI), which contain information on more than 100,000 Eukaryotic species. However, the submission of DNA sequences to these databases is accessible to all users and does not require verification of specimen identification. This failure to adhere to the standard guidelines set by taxonomically focused databases can lead to inaccuracies [648].

Users are inherently responsible for guaranteeing that databases contain only top-notch, uncontaminated sequences. A concept introduced by Tautz in 2003 suggested the creation of a database focused on taxonomy, allowing for advanced management techniques to preserve the credibility and traceability of data. This concept materialized in the form of the Barcode of Life Data System (BOLD), which serves as a collection exclusively for mtCOI barcoding sequences [649].

Significant research has been focused on the most common taxa of forensic interest, particularly within the families of Calliphoridae, Sarcophagidae, and Muscidae, as their DNA sequences dominate DNA databases. However, there has been limited attention given to less common taxa such as Muscidae, Phoridae, and Piophilidae, with only sparse datasets of sequences available for analysis. Therefore, it is essential to carefully consider and interpret molecular phylogenetic analysis in these cases. Wells and Stevens have provided a comprehensive examination of these specific aspects, highlighting the importance of the less explored areas of molecular analysis for species identification in forensic entomology [614].

Moreover, in aged cases, puparia frequently serve as the primary entomological evidence, with DNA analysis posing comparable difficulties to that of ancient DNA analysis, largely due to limited quantity, possible degradation, and the existence of PCR inhibitors [640].

Fragmentation and Chemical Modifications

The DNA extracted from aged and ancient materials may undergo extensive fragmentation. Various factors are responsible for the degradation of the double helix, either through natural processes or induced factors. The disintegration of cellular structures exposes the nuclear contents to degradation by both living and non-living environmental elements, including external nucleases released by microbial communities that decompose dead tissues. Exposure to ultraviolet light can also cause double-strand breaks in the DNA strands. In certain conditions like rapid drying and low temperatures, fragmentation could be minimized, but chemical alterations can occur, further destabilizing the DNA structure. Common forms of damage that contribute to DNA decay include oxidation of nitrogenous bases, hydrolytic deamination or depurination processes, and the formation of cross-links with other molecules. These damages can lead to the breaking of DNA strands or make them inaccessible to DNA polymerase during the PCR process [650- 662].

PCR Inhibition

PCR inhibition poses a significant obstacle in genetic analysis. Researchers often target mitochondrial genes like COI, COII, and 16S rDNA, which are present in large numbers per cell, as well as nuclear genes such as 18S rDNA and ITS2, which are organized as tandem-repeat sequences within the nuclear genome. Despite a high likelihood of success with this approach, external factors can still interfere with the amplification process. One common source of PCR inhibitors is contaminants that are co-extracted with the DNA, leading to impure samples if not properly purified. The exact molecular mechanism behind this inhibition is not fully understood, but it is theorized that these contaminants may form complexes with the DNA template or polymerases, preventing the enzyme from interacting with the substrate effectively [660].

Furthermore, certain compounds have the ability to chelate Mg^{+2}, a crucial cofactor for DNA polymerases. While it is challenging to predict the impact of inhibitors on environmental samples, a range of compounds that could be concurrently extracted with host DNA have been identified, including polysaccharides, humic and humic-like substances, other polyphenolic compounds, fulvic acids, and heavy metals. Notably, Pedersen and his colleagues have observed that humic acids attach to DNA molecules as a result of their negative surface charge, facilitating the formation of hindering molecular complexes. Interestingly, it is through the creation of such complexes that ancient DNA is able to endure over extended periods of time. To tackle this challenge in environmental sample analysis, the suggestion has been made to introduce substances like PVP (polyvinylpyrrolidone) or PVPP (polyvinylpolypyrrolidone) and BSA (bovine serum albumin) to PCR as a potential solution. These substances exhibit a stronger affinity for inhibitors compared to the reaction components that are effectively impeded (DNA template or DNA polymerases) [663, 664].

Chemical Identification of Puparia

In recent years, there has been a rise in alternative methodologies used for the identification of blowfly puparia species, deviating from the traditional morphological and DNA-based approaches. These new techniques focus on analyzing chemical profiles, which can be conveniently carried out using commonly available instruments within forensic laboratories. Notably, these chemical analyses offer a more objective perspective and are open to empirical validation, providing insights into their margin of error [665].

Among the array of proposed analytical methods, one particular approach has demonstrated considerable potential. This method entails the examination of organic compounds derived from the insect cuticle. The cuticle contains a diverse array of chemicals such as hydrocarbons, free fatty acids, alcohols, aldehydes, wax esters, and fatty acid methyl esters. These compounds serve various functions in the insect's physiology and life cycle [665].

Cuticular Hydrocarbons

Cuticular hydrocarbons (CHCs) are components of the lipid layer present on the exterior of insect cuticles. These compounds are comprised of extended chains of hydrogen and carbon atoms, typically ranging in length from C17 to C35. In insects, CHCs can be present in both saturated and unsaturated forms, and may also contain methyl groups [666]. Prior studies conducted on CHCs in different insect species have revealed their utility in serving as markers for identification and indicators of age [666].

Research conducted on blowflies that are crucial in forensic investigations has yielded encouraging findings. In particular, the utilization of Gas Chromatography-Mass Spectrometry (GC–MS) for analyzing Cuticular

Hydrocarbons (CHCs), non-metric multidimensional scaling analysis (NMDS), and permutational multivariate analysis of variance (PERMANOVA) for data analysis seems to be a reliable approach in distinguishing specimens in forensic cases across Europe [612]. Nevertheless, there are various barriers that impede the regular utilization of this methodology. These obstacles include the absence of an extensive repository containing the CHC signatures of fly puparia, fluctuations in these signatures over time that could impact identification accuracy, and the need for specialized and costly equipment, along with personnel training, leading to further challenges in its widespread implementation [613].

Lipids

Several studies indicate that flies have a wide range of fatty acids and sterols within them. Various types of free fatty acids have been detected, spanning from hexanoic acid (6:0) to hexacosanoic acid (26:0). However, most of these are present in minimal amounts in comparison to palmitic acid, palmitoleic acid, oleic acid, linoleic acid, and stearic acid. Similar to hydrocarbons, these lipids offer protection against dehydration, fungal invasion, and bacterial contamination [667, 668]. The chemical profiles can serve as a valuable resource for distinguishing and classifying at the puparium stage, as there are distinct variations both qualitatively and quantitatively among species. However, it is important to note that larvae and pupae possess unique chemical compositions, as do pupae at varying stages of development. While certain studies have showcased the ability of chemical profiles to differentiate between blowfly larvae and pupae in controlled laboratory settings, these same research findings have also illustrated that environmental factors like temperature, humidity, pupation surface, and diet significantly impact the precision of species identification through chemical analysis [669, 670].

Methodology Remarks

Some authors have emphasized the importance of conducting repeated molecular and morphological identifications of Diptera specimens in both larval and adult stages for forensic purposes, particularly when examining specimens from both recent and old cases. This practice is critical for the preservation of specimens housed in museum collections. Therefore, it is recommended that non-invasive methods for molecular and morphological analyses be given priority [671].

Proper preparation of specimens, such as employing dry mounting or preserving them in ethanol (70–95% at room temperature), along with utilizing immersion in DNA extraction buffers without damaging the specimens, are techniques that can be utilized to maintain the specimens for later analyses, particularly at the morphological level. Storing specimens at −20 °C may offer an optimal solution; however, this method is best suited for short-term storage or specific specimens, depending on the availability of freezing facilities and their consistent power supply. Storing specimens at −80 °C does not enhance specimen preservation and may impact DNA stability. The issue of reproducible molecular analysis might not be a concern when a large number of specimens are available, especially if they showcase unique diagnostic characteristics [671].

Application of Microbiome in Forensics

Microorganisms refer to minuscule beings like bacteria, fungi, viruses, algae, and certain small protozoa. The microbiome encompasses these microorganisms along with their environments and genetic material. Advancements in Next-Generation Sequencing (NGS) technology and bioinformatics have significantly enhanced the understanding of microbiomes in recent times. The microbiome plays a pivotal role in shaping human health, energy generation, agricultural practices, and environmental processes [672-674].

Over the past 15 years, numerous extensive initiatives have generated substantial volumes of data examining microbiomes in various environments worldwide, such as the Human Microbiome Project (HMP) and the Earth Microbiome Project (EMP). The HMP, initiated in October 2007, sought to investigate the composition and distribution of microbial communities in different regions of the human body while creating a repository of microbial genome sequences. It also aimed to elucidate the relationship between microbiology and human health. The EMP, launched in August 2010, aimed to establish a global repository of microbial diversity through a culture-independent methodology. The advancement of microbiome research into a new phase of rapid advancement has been propelled by a series of subsequent large-scale endeavors [675- 678].

In addition, various regions of the human body harbor distinct microbial populations. It is widely accepted that the microbial communities found in the oral cavity, skin, and gut are more varied compared to other areas of the body. The current research suggests that the microbiome in the environment does not adhere to the theory of 'everything is everywhere', but instead displays a biogeographic distribution. Significant differences in the composition of microbial communities can be observed among different geographical locations.

The widespread presence, diversity, and transferability of environmental microbiomes offer valuable insights into geographic patterns. Undoubtedly, these intriguing and significant discoveries demonstrate that forensic scientists can utilize microbiome analysis to address diverse challenges within the field of forensics [679-682].

Microorganisms have been utilized as evidence in forensic investigations since the late 19th century. Initially, the emphasis in microbial forensics was on examining the harmful effects and deadly potential of various microbes. The field of microbial forensics gained prominence as a result of the utilization of anthrax spores in letters as biological weapons in late 2001. Subsequently, microbial forensics was officially defined as the practice of utilizing scientific techniques to analyze evidence related to bioterrorism incidents, biocrimes, hoaxes, or accidental releases of biological agents or toxins, with the objective of identifying the responsible party [683- 685].

Before the introduction of Next Generation Sequencing (NGS) technology, forensic experts were unable to analyze microbes due to the sequencing methods needed to identify the microbiome being either time-consuming and expensive or reliant on culture-based techniques. With NGS technology, researchers can now swiftly and precisely identify the genetic sequences of all microorganisms present in a specimen, thus bypassing the risk of contamination and inaccuracies associated with microbial cultures. This advancement has proved to be valuable in forensic investigations [686- 688].

The initial scope of microbial forensics, originally limited to bioterrorism, has now evolved to encompass a broader range of potential applications in forensic science. It is now widely recognized that microbial forensics pertains to "the practice of analyzing microbiological evidence to generate leads in both criminal and civil investigations [685,690].

Recent advancements in microbiome technology have presented novel approaches to forensic investigations. One notable example is the utilization of the microbiome within the legal field to eliminate suspects and resolve criminal cases. In this discourse, they explore the recent progress in employing the microbiome for forensic purposes. Two primary techniques currently employed for microbiome characterization are amplicon sequencing and shotgun metagenomic sequencing. Amplicon sequencing, which focuses on specific marker genes or regions of interest, stands as the preferred Next-Generation Sequencing (NGS) method for forensic microbiome analysis. The most commonly used method involves amplicon sequencing of prokaryotic 16S ribosomal RNA (rRNA) genes and eukaryotic internal transcribed spacer (ITS) regions or 18S rRNA genes for microorganism profiling [691]. This method emphasizes high efficiency and cost-effectiveness by amplifying the 16/18S rRNA genes and the ITS regions. It is particularly well-suited for analyzing low-biomass samples without impacting host DNA. The Illumina MiSeq is the preferred tool for microbiome analysis, given its widespread use. To address its sequencing length limitations, this platform utilizes region-specific primers such as the V4 region of 16S rDNA and the V2 region of 18S rDNA. Consequently, precision at the genus level may be compromised and influenced by the selection of PCR cycles and primers. In contrast, long-read sequencing technologies like Oxford Nanopore Technologies (ONT) and Pacific Biosciences (PacBio) provide comprehensive solutions for full-length sequencing of hypervariable regions [692-694].

Modern databases must be updated to align with the most recent technological developments. In response, forensic scientists have utilized targeted sequencing techniques focused on microbial single nucleotide polymorphisms (SNPs) to analyze microbiomes. Researchers have utilized shotgun metagenomic datasets to pinpoint SNP markers accurately. In contrast to amplicon sequencing, shotgun metagenomic sequencing not only reveals taxonomic composition but also offers functional gene information and strain-level resolution. Nevertheless, this method comes with drawbacks, as it is more costly and less effective when dealing with specimens containing limited biomass or heavily contaminated by host genomes. As a result, the application of shotgun metagenomic sequencing in forensic investigations is restricted (Figure 36) [695, 696].

A forensic microbiome analysis pipeline has not yet been developed. Figure 20 demonstrates that pipelines similar to those utilized in other fields are employed in forensic microbiome analysis. The selection of a single sequence that reflects the characteristics of numerous sequences within a species has been implemented as a solution to this issue [673].

Two primary approaches for identifying suitable sequences as representatives involve grouping them into operational taxonomic units (OTUs) through clustering or refining them into amplicon sequence variants (ASVs) through denoising. Clustering sequences into OTUs is determined by a certain level of dissimilarity, typically set at 97% or 99% similarity. Generally, denoising techniques are favoured over clustering methods for amplicon analysis due to the higher accuracy of ASVs obtained from the denoising process. Key denoising algorithms include DADA2, Deblur, and UNOISE3 [697].

Several established amplicon analysis software packages, including Mothur, QIIME, QIIME2, USEARCH, and VSEARCH, offer clustering and denoising algorithms. The utilization of representative sequences enables the analysis of amplicon sequencing data even in the absence of taxonomic information [699-703]. Using a feature table (OTU/ASV table) without taxonomic details is generally not ideal for comparing different studies, as it requires repeating clustering or denoising each time new data is added. This method is not suitable for forensic applications or reference databases [703].

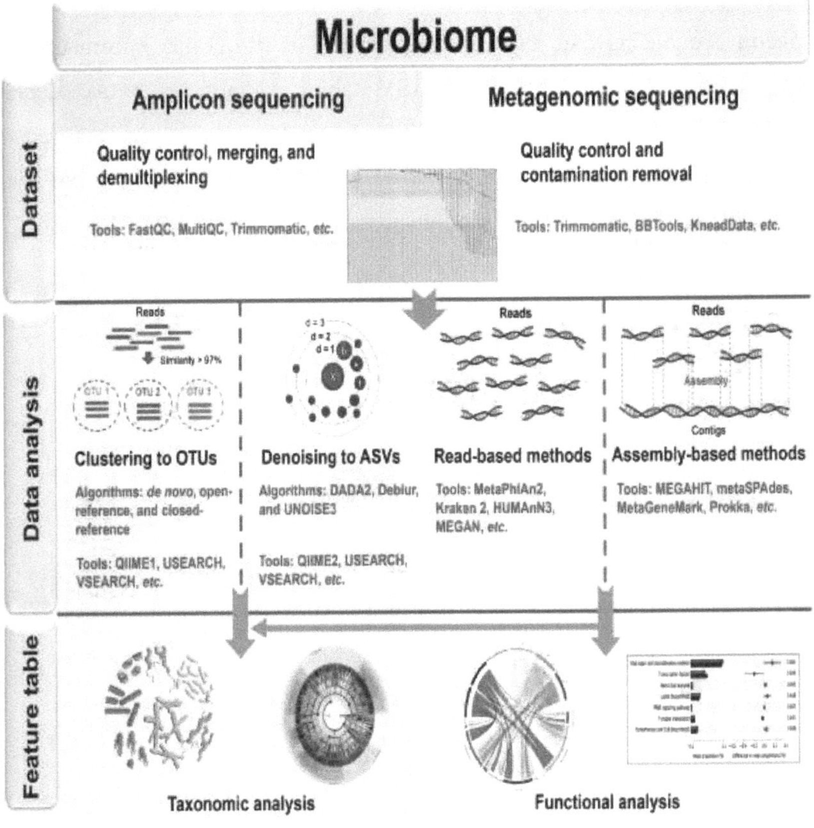

Figure 36: Illustrative visual representation showcasing the analytical processes for both amplicon sequencing and shotgun metagenomic sequencing. OTU refers to the operational taxonomic unit, while ASV stands for the amplicon sequence variant [703].

The table featuring taxonomic information such as kingdom, phylum, class, order, family, genus, and species offers a more user-friendly experience. Various public databases like SILVA, Greengenes, and UNITE can be accessed for taxonomic references. Shotgun metagenomic sequencing has the capability to provide detailed functional information and enhanced taxonomic annotation. However, the growing volume of data necessitates additional computational resources and bioinformatics expertise, which can limit the application of metagenomic sequencing in forensic investigations. Despite this limitation, shotgun metagenomic sequencing is able to accurately identify all DNA fragments present in a sample, including both microbial and host DNA [704-707].

Prior to conducting taxonomic and functional analyses, it is essential to ensure quality control and eliminate contaminants from the raw data. Popular tools such as KneadData, Trimmomatic, and BBTools (http://sourceforge.net/projects/ bbmap) are commonly employed for this purpose. There are two main approaches for performing taxonomic and functional analyses: one involves aligning clean sequences with databases (read-based methods), while the other involves assembling reads into contigs (assembly-based methods). MetaPhlAn2, Kraken 2, HUMAnN3, and MEGAN are frequently utilized for taxonomic and functional profiling using read-based methods. The reads can be compiled into contigs using MEGAHIT or metaSPAdes [708- 716].

Afterwards, the compiled contigs are distinguished using either MetaGene-Mark or Prokka. Metagenomic research utilizing assembly methods is notably uncommon in the field of forensics. Additionally, individuals in the forensic science community appear to place a higher emphasis on taxonomic data rather than functional data [717, 718].

Application in forensics

Significant advancements in microbiome research methodologies, specifically those utilizing next-generation sequencing (NGS) technology, have led to an enhanced emphasis on microbiome analysis for forensic purposes. Examination of microbiome data, such as amplicon and metagenome sequencing information, offers multiple benefits in the realm of forensics, including but not limited to individual identification, geolocation determination, estimation of post-mortem interval (PMI), and additional applications (refer to Figure 37 for illustration) [719, 720].

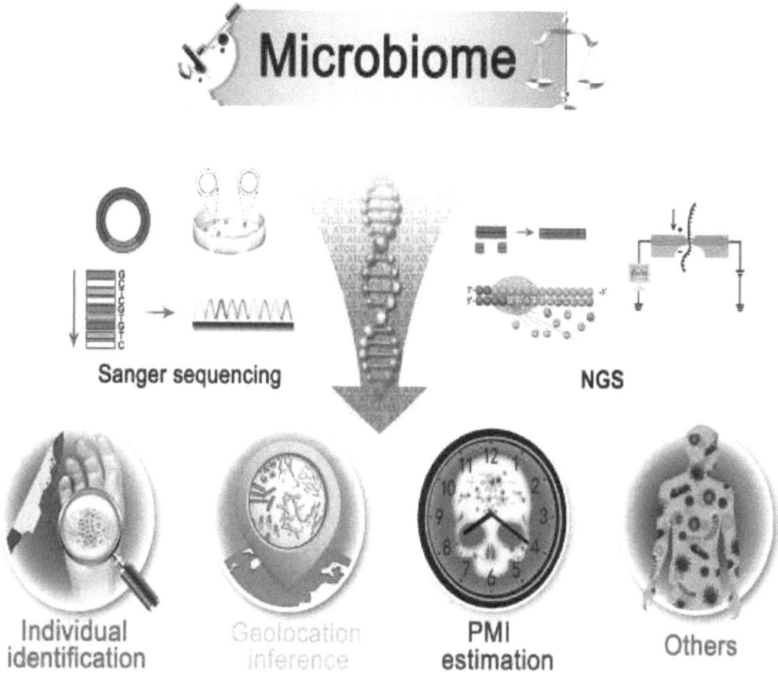

Figure 37: Compared to Sanger sequencing, forensic analysis using metagenomics has significantly decreased the sequencing cost while enhancing throughput and read length with the advent of NGS technology. This has propelled forensic science into a new era of advancement. The microbiome has the potential to impact various aspects of forensics, such as personal identification, geolocation inference, and post-mortem interval estimation. Furthermore, beyond the mentioned uses, the microbiome could lead to advancements in forensic pathology, toxicology, and testing for substance abuse. Consequently, progress in metagenomics is poised to offer fresh perspectives in the realm of forensic applications. NGS refers to next-generation sequencing while PMI stands for post-mortem interval [720].

Individual identification

Genotyping short tandem repeats (STRs) through the utilization of polymerase chain reaction (PCR) and capillary electrophoresis (CE) stands as the cornerstone of forensic DNA analysis and finds extensive application in individual identification and paternity testing. Challenges in forensic casework often arise from the diminution or insufficiency of DNA samples, rendering further analysis unfeasible. However, microorganisms can offer vital clues to aid investigators. Recent research indicates that the quantity of microbial cells present in the human body exceeds the total number of human cells by a factor of 1.3. A human microbiota harbours in excess of one million genes, a magnitude approximately 500 times greater than the number of genes present in the human genome [721- 724].

The makeup of microbial communities in an individual is intricately shaped by a combination of genetic predisposition, environmental surroundings, and the habits and behaviors of the host. It is believed that each individual harbours a distinct and specific collection of microorganisms that can be detected and characterized through the analysis of their microbiome [675].

Researchers from Harvard University conducted an analysis of the microbiomes present in saliva, skin, faeces, and other bodily locations of 242 participants in the Human Microbiome Project. The purpose of the study was to assess the distinctiveness and consistency of microbial communities in order to identify individuals. The findings revealed that specific microbial characteristics linked to humans were effective in distinguishing one person from another. Moreover, genetic features were found to be more resistant to change over time compared to taxonomic features. Approximately 30% of individuals could still be accurately identified between 30 and 300 days later using genetic analysis of a typical bodily site, with minimal false positive results. The study concluded that microbiomes found in faeces exhibited the highest level of stability, with over 80% of individuals remaining identifiable even after one year. Conversely, microbiomes in skin and vaginal regions were more susceptible to external influences that could alter their composition [726].

Microbiomes present on bodily surfaces, such as the skin and hair, may have a significant impact on forensic investigations, as individuals can easily transfer their microbiota to other individuals or objects through touch. The presence of individuals in a shared living environment can influence the microbial community on their skin, leading to similarities in skin microbiomes among cohabitating individuals due to frequent physical contact and shared surfaces within the household. The transfer of skin microbiomes between individuals who do not live together could also serve as valuable trace evidence. A study conducted by Williams and Gibson demonstrated the potential to identify sexual contact through the analysis of microbiomes from the pubic region, as the unique composition of pubic microbiomes can distinguish one individual from another. In cases of sexual assault, it was found that more than 10% of the pubic microbiome in women was derived from the assailant, highlighting the forensic significance of microbiome analysis. By identifying the assailant, it is possible to determine if sexual contact has taken place based on microbiome analysis. Furthermore, the human microbiome is not only transferred between individuals but also persists on objects that have been touched. Research has shown differences in the bacterial populations found on people's hands compared to those present on personal objects such as computers and smartphones [727- 731].

A significant connection was observed between the microbial makeup present on individuals' hands and that found on the screens of their electronic devices. Inanimate surfaces have the ability to host these bacteria for a period exceeding two weeks. Personal behavior can have a significant impact on the microbial composition in one's surroundings. As an example, the bacteria on a kitchen counter can quickly come to resemble that of the homeowner after moving into a new residence. Each person has the potential to create a unique 'microbial cloud' by releasing microbes into the environment. Through metagenomic analysis, most individuals can be distinguished based on the composition of this 'microbial cloud [732]. It is feasible to distinguish an individual by examining the environmental microbiome overall. Research focusing on the body surface microbiome for individual identification typically utilizes amplicon sequencing of the 16S rRNA genes. However, this approach is limited in its ability to differentiate between species and strains. In a study conducted by Schmedes *et al.*, the nucleotide diversity of shotgun metagenomes from skin microbiomes (collected from 12 individuals and 17 skin body sites at three different time intervals spanning over 2.5 years) was recognized as a potential marker for individual identification. Subsequently, they introduced hidSkinPlex, a targeted sequencing panel that incorporates clade-specific markers derived from skin microbiomes to distinguish between individuals [733].

Skin microbiome compositions from different regions of the body such as the foot, hand, and manubrium were identified with a high degree of precision, ranging from 92% to 100%. Furthermore, enhancements were made to the marker set known as hidSkinPlex+, comprising 365 SNPs from 135 markers. This refined marker set, although smaller in size, boasts increased resilience compared to the initial version and maintains its ability to effectively pinpoint individuals, as evidenced by a Matthews correlation coefficient of 0.949 [733- 735].

Additionally, the history of bacterial infections can be retraced by utilizing clustered regularly interspaced short palindromic repeats (CRISPRs). The focused sequencing of bacterial CRISPR spacers offers more detailed phylogenetic information compared to other markers. According to research conducted by Toyomane et al., the analysis of 24 potential CRISPR arrays from a shotgun metagenome dataset of human skin was used to establish uniqueness. The outcomes indicated a significant polymorphism of CRISPR spacers within the skin microbiome. CRISPR typing exhibited a superior accuracy rate (95.2%) in contrast to 16S rRNA gene sequencing (52.6%) [736, 737].

Further research is necessary to delineate the unique characteristics of the body surface microbiome on a genetic level. The process of distinguishing individuals based on their body surface microbiome poses challenges in forensic analysis. In a study conducted by Wilkins *et al.*, samples of skin and household surface microbiota were gathered throughout four seasons to assess the consistency of connecting individuals to their respective living environments over extended periods. The study revealed a decrease in accuracy as the time gap between skin and household surface samples increased. A majority of operational taxonomic units (OTUs) were found to persist on skin or household surfaces for less than a full season. Additionally, findings from another study highlighted how fluctuations in the human skin microbiome throughout the day could also impact the reliability of identifying individuals based on their microbiome [738, 739].

At all sampling locations, a noteworthy shift in the relative abundance of 160 species was observed between morning and evening. These findings indicate the importance of taking into account the temporal decay of microbiota traces and diurnal patterns of microbiota when developing the skin microbiome as a possible forensic tool for individual identification [721].

Geolocation inference

In the realm of forensic investigation, analysis of environmental samples such as soil, water, and vegetation can yield valuable insights. Examining soil can offer crucial evidence in pinpointing suspects and crime scenes, as well as providing guidance in resolving cases. Research in environmental microbiology has revealed a diverse array of microorganisms that are commonly found in water and soil, with variations in species and strains depending on the geographical location. The specific microbiological data associated with a particular location could suggest recent relocation by an individual. Advancements in molecular biology and metagenomic technology have led to a deeper understanding of microbial distribution patterns, thereby enhancing the utilization of microbiome-based analysis for location inference [740- 742].

Forensic geolocation has previously been examined through the utilization of terminal restriction fragment length polymorphism (TRFLP) and denaturing gel electrophoresis (DGGE). Habtom *et al.* has employed TRFLP in recent studies to analyze soil microbial DNA profiles at various geographic scales ranging from local to regional levels (2 m– 260 km). Their findings indicate that soil microbial DNA profiles can provide insights into the geographical origin of a sample with a resolution as fine as 25 meters [743- 745].

Various molecular techniques were applied in microbiology to determine geolocation, such as TRFLP, ribosomal intergenic spacer analysis (RISA), microarrays, and NGS (Roche 454, Ion Torrent, and Illumina MiSeq), along with n-alkanes and fatty alcohol profiles. The study revealed that TRFLP and Illumina

MiSeq were the most effective methods for 16S rRNA gene sequencing and RISA. Demane`che *et al.* conducted a blinded test to assess the reliability of soil bacterial communities for forensic analysis. Two biological techniques, RISA and 16S rRNA gene sequencing, were used to differentiate soil bacterial communities successfully, with single-source soil identification achieved using either method. However, a combined approach of both methods was needed for characterizing mixed-source soil samples. In a separate investigation, Yang *et al.* performed 16S rRNA gene sequencing on soil samples from 529 locations across 61 districts in 10 major cities in China. Bacterial community analysis allowed for accurate assignment of random soil samples to specific districts and cities with 66.7% and 90% accuracy, respectively [746-748]. This research has demonstrated that soil microorganisms have the potential to offer insights into the origins of unidentified samples and enable the comparison of samples obtained from suspects or crime scenes. The majority of studies on geolocation inference have focused on the bacterial community present in the soil. It is worth noting that soil harbors a rich diversity of microflora including bacteria, fungi, protozoa, and viral fauna, among others. Lilje *et al.* conducted a study on various microbial communities to establish guidelines for the management of soil metagenomic data and database retrieval for forensic purposes. The sequencing data utilized in the research encompassed the 18S rRNA genes of fungi, the small subunit ribosomal RNA (SSU rRNA) regions of arbuscular mycorrhizal fungi (AMF), and the 16S rRNA genes of bacteria. Various methods were employed for data filtration in the data management process. A comparison of the data indicated that the creation and utilization of a filtered 18S rRNA database could significantly enhance computational efficiency and flexibility [749].

Giampaoli and colleagues employed a metabarcoding technique to effectively, precisely, and sensitively examine the genetic composition of specific soils, including microflora, plant, metazoan, and protozoan DNA. The utilization of DNA metabarcoding proves to be a beneficial method for distinguishing microbial components in samples that share similar geological backgrounds but originate from varying environments. By utilizing shotgun metagenomic sequencing, the complete microflora, encompassing bacteria, fungi, and viruses, among others, can be simultaneously identified in a given sample. Consequently, metagenomics emerges as a valuable tool for deducing geolocation within the realm of forensic analytics. Danko and team compiled a comprehensive global atlas comprising 4758 metagenomic samples gathered across 60 cities worldwide over a span of three years [750, 751].

Future perspectives

In order to establish a regional database of forensic entomofauna, a thorough investigation into the decay patterns of corpses and the succession waves of insects is essential across various climatic zones, seasons, and habitats. Specific research is required to analyze the impact of temperature, relative humidity, rainfall, and other factors on the developmental stages of forensic insects, in order to create a comprehensive maturation scale for each insect species [749].

Securing funding and financial support from research and development agencies is crucial for the collection of accurate crime scene data, simulation site data, and the identification of molecular markers to distinguish between different insect species. It is imperative for forensic entomologists to conduct routine forensic entomological assessments at crime scenes to advance scientific and technological progress in the field [750].

Artificial Intelligence in the Field of Forensic Biology

Since DNA breaks down rapidly over time, there is very little DNA left at crime scenes, but microbes are ubiquitous in both natural and manmade environments due to their rule of development. The use of microbes as legally admissible criminal evidence is very promising. Additionally, the development of high-throughput sequencing technology and enhanced analytical platforms has made it possible for forensics to employ microbial traces from crime scenes or the human body to solve crimes. As a result, the field of forensic microbiology—also referred to as the microbiology of death—was born. Numerous forensic science issues, including determining the cause of death and biological crime, identifying specific individuals, and estimating the post-mortem interval (PMI) and place of death, have been resolved by microbiomes . In forensic microbiology, there are still a lot of unanswered questions, though: What is the impact of external and internal influences on microbial changes? What microbes are suitable for use as biomarkers in forensic medicine applications? Which microorganisms follow the law of co-succession after death? [752, 753].

The use of AI in forensic microbiology will concentrate on the following areas: novel insights and advancements in AI methods for microbial solutions to forensic issues; use of AI in data processing model development, algorithm creation and optimization, and forensic microbiology; enhancement of forensic science techniques for microbial DNA sampling and other analysis processes using AI algorithms; In order to use AI techniques to address pertinent forensic problems, the use of microbiome combines with transcriptome, proteome, metabolomics, and other multi-omics methodologies.An essential field for criminal investigations is forensic medicine and toxicology, which has enormous potential for advancement with the aid of artificial intelligence. There are numerous drawbacks to the conventional autopsy and opinion-forming process, which AI can help to address. AI will be crucial in framing the various opinions of medicolegal importance in a number of forensic medicine procedures, such as the analysis of toxins, the collection of various samples of medicolegal importance from the body cavity, the detection of pathological changes in various organs of the body, the detection of various stains on the body, the detection of a weapon used in the crime, time since death calculations, etc. [753, 754]. Artificial Intelligence techniques have advanced rapidly in recent years. The goal of AI, a subfield of computer science, is to mimic the intelligent behaviour of people or animals to learn new things, improve algorithms, make judgments, or forecast the future. Numerous scientific and technical domains, including machine vision, pattern recognition, medical image analysis, and natural language processing, have made use of it. AI's potent skills have now been applied to forensic microbiology to help legal medical professionals in their day-to-day jobs and, consequently, to improve the usage of microorganisms in the field of forensic medicine to solve difficulties. AI methods will present a fresh and promising opportunity for forensic microbiology. PCR technology takes a lengthy time to finish the experiment, although being more sophisticated than conventional biochemical and microbiological techniques. Furthermore, the incorporation and use of AI technology has the potential to completely transform the identification and management of bacteria in addition to optimizing the current procedure (Figure 38) [755].

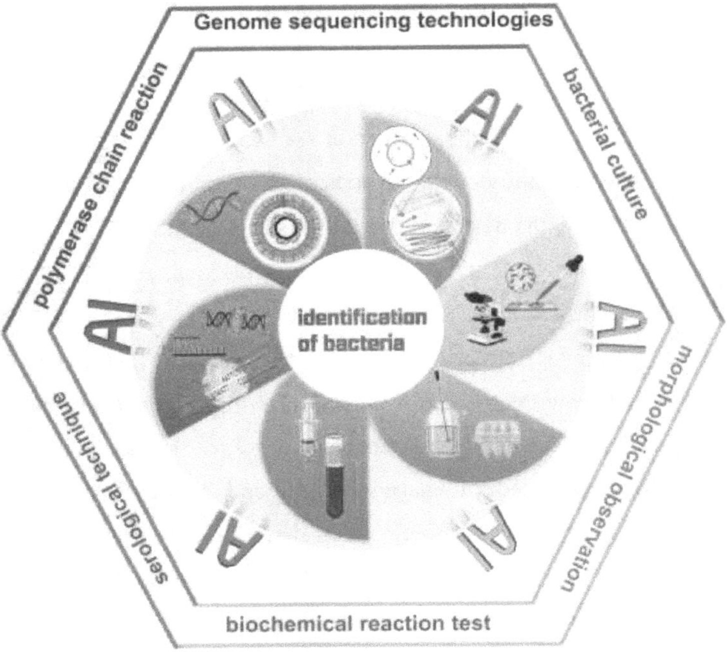

Figure 38: The detection of infectious bacterial infections is made easier by artificial intelligence [755]

Conclusions

The investigation of the microbiome holds significant promise for the field of forensic sciences, although it faces a number of challenges. One of the primary issues involves ensuring the stability, reproducibility, and sensitivity of bacterial analysis. While microbiome analysis is frequently utilized in the realms of medicine and public health, its application in forensic science is more complex due to uncertainties regarding the abundance of bacterial communities present in samples. Furthermore, the preservation of samples is a point of contention, as factors such as storage temperature and duration can impact the quality of extraction and the identification of bacterial communities. Another obstacle is the fluctuation of an individual's microbiome over time and across different body locations.

In order to address these issues, the field of futures studies needs to develop protocols for research inquiries, such as sampling techniques, sample sizes, storage procedures, limitations, and criteria for monitoring and controlling variables. It is crucial to identify the typical bacterial populations found on substrates and surfaces, and those that could potentially contaminate samples. Adequate amounts of bacterial DNA must be collected during sampling to accurately assess the microbiome, or at the very least, the predominant phyla or classes of bacteria that are unique to fluids or tissues. [836].

NGS technology, which is commonly utilized in forensic laboratories for human genetic investigations by companies like Illumina, Thermo Scientific, Qiagen, and Roche, needs to be further developed for microbiota analysis. This requires specialized expertise in bioinformatics analysis and the adaptation of appropriate kits and protocols due to the limited availability of bacterial DNA.

Despite being relatively costly, ranging from $285 to $500 per sample, additional research is necessary to fully establish the potential of this approach.

Furthermore, the results of microbiota analysis must be tailored for legal proceedings to ensure clarity and eliminate any doubts in court. The question of evidence is a crucial aspect in criminal cases, particularly in the assessment of evidence by judges and juries within the framework of French criminal law. Their personal conviction is formed through an analytical evaluation of the evidence, making it a key procedural element in legitimizing criminal decisions. The outcome of a criminal trial is heavily influenced by the presence and quality of evidence, which is evaluated based on its legality as well as scientific parameters such as integrity, accuracy, and reliability. The admissibility of results depends on adherence to specific conditions, including the involvement of authorized and qualified individuals in the analysis process. [143].

At a crime scene, there is an increasing amount of biological evidence that may be exploited, although not all may be linked directly to the crime at hand. Evaluating the relevance of such traces is crucial in forming a scientific conclusion.

In order to utilize microbial data effectively in forensics, innovative methods of classification need to be developed, taking into consideration various limitations such as human microbiome diversity, data errors in classification, environmental variables, and genetic factors.

The analysis of microbiological evidence in forensics involves comparing samples of evidence with known microorganisms.

To establish the microbiome as a valid form of evidence, rigorous statistical techniques must be validated to ensure accuracy, particularly in accounting for the various factors influencing microbiome composition.

It is crucial to consider the future implications of utilizing the microbiome in forensic sciences, as these studies can provide valuable insights into individual health and lifestyle. Establishing a legal framework for the use of bacterial data, similar to genetic markers in DNA analysis regulated by the criminal procedure code, will be imperative.

A total of 340 adult insects were recovered from a decomposing rabbit carcass, predominantly comprising flies. The highest numbers and greatest species diversity of flies were observed during the early stages of decomposition, with a high prevalence of various pathogenic bacteria in these flies. The presence of infective bacteria such as *E. coli*, *Klebsiella pneumoniae*, *Pseudomonas aeruginosa*, and *Proteus mirabilis* within the studied flies may contribute to current public health challenges worldwide.

Flies, due to their behavior and frequent contact with waste, carcasses, and food, act as mechanical vectors for transferring harmful agents. Hence, it is imperative for the government to raise awareness about personal hygiene, clean surfaces prone to fly contact, and prevent cross-contamination to mitigate bacterial infections.

In criminal investigations, the significant role of entomofauna as silent witnesses is increasingly being recognized by police investigators, medico-legal experts, and forensic investigators. Forensic entomology, once disregarded, has now emerged as a crucial scientific tool in crime scene investigations, aided by advancements in scientific research and technology. Expert forensic entomologists are now employed by law enforcement agencies worldwide to provide valuable insights into crime cases.

Proficiency in regional entomofauna, insect biology, and taxonomy is essential for effectively utilizing forensic entomofauna as indicators in crime investigations. Adequate education and training for personnel collecting insects and biological samples at crime scenes are crucial, as the quality of evidence gathered directly impacts the interpretation by forensic entomologists and the judiciary.

Given the challenges in identifying immature Diptera in forensic entomology, combining different methods after evaluating their efficacy and limitations is recommended. Prioritizing non-invasive analysis protocols and technology is also necessary, along with the creation of lab databases containing local species for enhanced DNA sequence comparisons. While chemical cuticular analyses are valuable in forensic entomology, the specialized equipment and expertise required pose constraints on widespread adoption in forensic laboratories

References

1. Kamaluddin, M., Shariff, N. & Matsaat, G. Mechanical profiles of murder and murderers: An extensive review. *Malays. J. Pathol.* **40**, 10 (2018).
2. Junkins, E. N. & Carter, D. O. Relationships between Human Remains, Graves and the Depositional Environment. In *Taphonomy of Human Remains: Forensic Analysis of the Dead and the Depositional Environment* (eds Schotsmans, E. M. J., Márquez-Grant, N. & Forbes, S. L.) 143–154, https://doi.org/10.1002/9781118953358.ch11 (John Wiley & Sons, Ltd, 2017).
3. Bergeret, L.-F.-É. *Infanticide, momification naturelle du cadavre*. (Arbois: impr. de E. Javel, 1864).
4. Smith, K. G. *A manual of forensic entomology*. (Trustees of the British Museum, 1986).
5. Anderson, G. S. Determining time of death using blow fly eggs in the early postmortem interval. *Int. J. Legal Med.* **118** (2004).
6. Anderson, G. S. Comparison of decomposition rates and faunal colonization of carrion in indoor and outdoor environments: decomposition rates and faunal colonization of carrion. *J. Forensic Sci.* **56**, 136–142 (2011).
7. Bharti, M. & Singh, D. Insect Faunal Succession on Decaying Rabbit Carcasses in Punjab, India. *J. Forensic Sci.* **48**, 2001358 (2003).
8. Carter, D. O., Yellowlees, D. & Tibbett, M. Cadaver decomposition in terrestrial ecosystems. *Naturwissenschaften* **94**, 12–24 (2006).
9. Benbow, M. E., Lewis, A. J., Tomberlin, J. K. & Pechal, J. L. Seasonal Necrophagous Insect Community Assembly During Vertebrate Carrion Decomposition. *J. Med. Entomol.* **50**, 440–450 (2013).

10. Finley, S. J., Benbow, M. E. & Javan, G. T. Microbial communities associated with human decomposition and their potential use as postmortem clocks. *Int. J. Legal Med.* **129**, 623–632 (2015).
11. Metcalf, J. L. *et al.* Microbial community assembly and metabolic function during mammalian corpse decomposition. *Science* **351**, 158–162 (2016).
12. Carter, D. O. & Tibbett, M. Does repeated burial of skeletal muscle tissue (Ovis aries) in soil affect subsequent decomposition? *Appl. Soil Ecol.* **40**, 529–535 (2008).
13. Gunn, A. & Bird, J. The ability of the blowflies Calliphora vomitoria (Linnaeus), Calliphora vicina (Rob-Desvoidy) and Lucilia sericata (Meigen) (Diptera: Calliphoridae) and the muscid flies Muscina stabulans (Fallén) and Muscina prolapsa (Harris) (Diptera: Muscidae) to colonise buried remains. *Forensic Sci. Int.* **207**, 198–204 (2011).
14. Gunn, A. The colonisation of remains by the muscid flies Muscina stabulans (Fallén) and Muscina prolapsa (Harris) (Diptera: Muscidae). *Forensic Sci. Int.* **266**, 349–356 (2016).
15. Janaway, R. The preservation of organic materials in association with metal artefacts deposited in inhumation graves. In *Death, decay and reconstruction: approaches to archaeology and forensic science* (eds Boddington, A., Garland, A. & Janaway, R.) 127–141 (Manchester University Press, 1987).
16. Janaway, R. The decay of buried human remains and their associated materials. In *Studies in crime: an introduction to forensic archaeology* (eds Hunter, J., Roberts, C. & Martin, A.) 58–85 (Routledge, 1996).

17. Janaway, R. C., Percival, S. L. & Wilson, A. S. Decomposition of Human Remains. In *Microbiology and Aging* (ed. Percival, S. L.) 313–334, https://doi.org/10.1007/978-1-59745-327-1_14 (Humana Press, 2009).

18. Szpila, K., Voss, J. G. & Pape, T. A new dipteran forensic indicator in buried bodies. *Med. Vet. Entomol.* https://doi.org/10.1111/j.1365-2915.2010.00883.x (2010).

19. Carter, D. O., Yellowlees, D. & Tibbett, M. Moisture can be the dominant environmental parameter governing cadaver decomposition in soil. *Forensic Sci. Int.* **200**, 60–66 (2010).

20. Mariani, R., García-Mancuso, R., Varela, G. L. & Inda, A. M. Entomofauna of a buried body: Study of the exhumation of a human cadaver in Buenos Aires, Argentina. *Forensic Sci. Int.* **237**, 19–26 (2014).

21. Motter, M. G. A Contribution to the Study of the Fauna of the Grave. A Study of on Hundred and Fifty Disinterments, with Some Additional Experimental Observations. *J. N. Y. Entomol. Soc.* **6**, 201–231 (1898).

22. Lord, W. D., Adkins, T. R. & Catts, E. P. Use of Synthesiomyia nudesita (Van Der Wulp) (Diptera: Muscidae) and Calliphora vicina (Robineau-Desvoidy) (Diptera: Calliphoridae) to estimate the time of death of a body buried under a house. *J. Agric. Entomol.* (1992).

23. Rodriguez, W. C. & Bass, W. M. Decomposition of buried bodies and methods that may aid in their location. *J. Forensic Sci.* **30**, 836–852 (1985).

24. Rysavy, N. M. & Goff, M. L. Preliminary Observations of Arthropods Associated with Buried Carrion on Oahu. *J. Forensic Sci.* **60**, 462–467 (2015).

25. Finley, S. J., Pechal, J. L., Benbow, M. E., Robertson, B. K. & Javan, G. T. Microbial Signatures of Cadaver Gravesoil During Decomposition. *Microb. Ecol.* **71**, 524–529 (2016).
26. VanLaerhoven, S. L. & Anderson, G. S. Insect succession on buried carrion in two biogeoclimatic zones of British Columbia. *J. Forensic Sci.* **44**, 32–43 (1999).
27. Lowe, A. C. *et al.* The effect of soil texture on the degradation of textiles associated with buried bodies. *Forensic Sci. Int.* **231**, 331–339 (2013).
28. Bernhardt, V. *et al.* Muscina prolapsa (Harris 1780): Ein bislang unterschätztes Werkzeug der forensischen Entomologie. *Rechtsmedizin* **26**, 97–102 (2016).
29. Marais-Werner, A., Myburgh, J., Meyer, A., Nienaber, W. & Steyn, M. Decomposition patterns of buried remains at different intervals in the Central Highveld region of South Africa. *Med. Sci. Law* **57**, 115–123 (2017).
30. Gaudry, E. The Insects Colonisation of Buried Remains. In *Current Concepts in Forensic Entomology* (eds Amendt, J., Goff, M. L., Campobasso, C. P. & Grassberger, M.) 273–311, https://doi.org/10.1007/978-1-4020-9684-6_13 (Springer Netherlands, 2010).
31. Pechal, J. L. *et al.* Microbial Community Functional Change during Vertebrate Carrion Decomposition. *PLoS ONE* **8**, e79035 (2013).
32. Finley, S. J., Benbow, M. E. & Javan, G. T. Potential applications of soil microbial ecology and next-generation sequencing in criminal investigations. *Appl. Soil Ecol.* **88**, 69–78 (2015).
33. Goff, M. L. Early Postmortem Changes and Stages of Decomposition. In *Current Concepts in Forensic Entomology* (eds Amendt, J., Goff, M. L.,

Campobasso, C. P. & Grassberger, M.) 1–24, https://doi.org/10.1007/978-1-4020-9684-6_1 (Springer Netherlands, 2009).
34. Wilson, A. S. *et al.* Modelling the buried human body environment in upland climes using three contrasting field sites. *Forensic Sci. Int.* **169**, 6–18 (2007).
35. Haglund, W. D. & Sorg, M. H. *Forensic taphonomy: the postmortem fate of human remains*. (CRC Press, 1997).
36. Forbes, S. L. Potential determinants of postmortem and post burial interval of buried remains. In *Soil analysis in forensic taphonomy* (eds Tibbett, M. & Carter, D. O.) 225–246 (CRC Press, 2008).
37. Payne, J. A., King, E. W. & Beinhart, G. Arthropod Succession and Decomposition of Buried Pigs. *Nature* **219**, 1180–1181 (1968).
38. Rodriguez, W. C. & Bass, W. M. Insect Activity and its Relationship to Decay Rates of Human Cadavers in East Tennessee. *J. Forensic Sci.* **28**, 11524J (1983).
39. Bourel, B., Tournel, G., Hedouin, V. & Gosset, D. Entomofauna of buried bodies in northern France. *Int. J. Legal Med.* **118** (2004).
40. Pechal, J. L. *et al.* The potential use of bacterial community succession in forensics as described by high throughput metagenomic sequencing. *Int. J. Legal Med.* **128**, 193–205 (2014).
41. Hyde, E. R., Haarmann, D. P., Lynne, A. M., Bucheli, S. R. & Petrosino, J. F. The Living Dead: Bacterial Community Structure of a Cadaver at the Onset and End of the Bloat Stage of Decomposition. *PLoS ONE* **8**, e77733 (2013).
42. Hyde, E. R., Haarmann, D. P., Petrosino, J. F., Lynne, A. M. & Bucheli, S. R. Initial insights into bacterial succession during human decomposition. *Int. J. Legal Med.* **129**, 661–671 (2015).

43. Carter, D. O., Metcalf, J. L., Bibat, A. & Knight, R. Seasonal variation of postmortem microbial communities. *Forensic Sci. Med. Pathol.* **11**, 202–207 (2015).
44. Javan, G. T., Finley, S. J., Abidin, Z. & Mulle, J. G. The Thanatomicrobiome: A Missing Piece of the Microbial Puzzle of Death. *Front. Microbiol.* **7** (2016).
45. Guo, J. *et al.* Potential use of bacterial community succession for estimating post-mortem interval as revealed by high-throughput sequencing. *Sci. Rep.* **6** (2016).
46. Chimutsa, M., Olakanye, A. O., Thompson, T. J. U. & Ralebitso-Senior, T. K. Soil fungal community shift evaluation as a potential cadaver decomposition indicator. *Forensic Sci. Int.* **257**, 155–159 (2015).
47. Cobaugh, K. L., Schaeffer, S. M. & DeBruyn, J. M. Functional and Structural Succession of Soil Microbial Communities below Decomposing Human Cadavers. *PLOS ONE* **10**, e0130201 (2015).
48. Metcalf, J. L. *et al.* A microbial clock provides an accurate estimate of the postmortem interval in a mouse model system. *eLife* **2** (2013).
49. Weatherbee, C. R., Pechal, J. L., Stamper, T. & Benbow, M. E. Post-Colonization Interval Estimates Using Multi-Species Calliphoridae Larval Masses and Spatially Distinct Temperature Data Sets: A Case Study. *Insects* **8**, 40 (2017).
50. Hauther, K. A., Cobaugh, K. L., Jantz, L. M., Sparer, T. E. & DeBruyn, J. M. Estimating Time Since Death from Postmortem Human Gut Microbial Communities. *J. Forensic Sci.* **60**, 1234–1240 (2015).

51. Santo Domingo, J. W., Siefring, S. C. & Haugland, R. A. Real-time PCR method to detect Enterococcus faecalis in water. *Biotechnol. Lett.* **25**, 261–265 (2003).
52. Guo, X. *et al.* Development of a real-time PCR method for Firmicutes and Bacteroidetes in faeces and its application to quantify intestinal population of obese and lean pigs. *Lett. Appl. Microbiol.* **47**, 367–373 (2008).
53. Hermann-Bank, M., Skovgaard, K., Stockmarr, A., Larsen, N. & Mølbak, L. The Gut Microbiotassay: a high-throughput qPCR approach combinable with next generation sequencing to study gut microbial diversity. *BMC Genomics* **14**, 788 (2013).
54. Veskoukis, A. S. *et al.* Effects of xanthine oxidase inhibition on oxidative stress and swimming performance in rats. *Appl. Physiol. Nutr. Metab. Physiol. Appl. Nutr. Metab.* **33**, 1140–1154 (2008).
55. Booth, F. W. & Laye, M. J. Lack of adequate appreciation of physical exercise's complexities can pre-empt appropriate design and interpretation in scientific discovery. *J. Physiol.* **587**, 5527–5539 (2009).
56. Nikolaidis, M. G. *et al.* Effect of chronic wheel running on the fatty acid composition of phospholipids and triacylglycerols in rat serum, skeletal muscle and heart. *Acta Physiol. Scand.* **181**, 199–208 (2004).
57. Allen, D. G., Lamb, G. D. & Westerblad, H. Skeletal muscle fatigue: cellular mechanisms. *Physiol. Rev.* **88**, 287–332 (2008).
58. Kyparos, A., Feeback, D. L., Layne, C. S., Martinez, D. A. & Clarke, M. S. F. Mechanical stimulation of the plantar foot surface attenuates soleus muscle atrophy induced by hindlimb unloading in rats. *J. Appl. Physiol. Bethesda Md 1985* **99**, 739–746 (2005).

59. Röckl, K. S. C., Witczak, C. A. & Goodyear, L. J. Signaling mechanisms in skeletal muscle: acute responses and chronic adaptations to exercise. *IUBMB Life* **60**, 145–153 (2008).

60. Carter, D. O., Yellowlees, D. & Tibbett, M. Temperature affects microbial decomposition of cadavers (Rattus rattus) in contrasting soils. *Appl. Soil Ecol.* **40**, 129–137 (2008).

61. Roux C., Talbot-Wright B., Robertson J., Crispino F., Ribaux O. The end of the (forensic science) world as we know it? The example of trace evidence. Philos. *Trans. R. Soc. Lond. B Biol. Sci.* 2015; 370:20140260. doi: 10.1098/rstb.2014.0260.

62. Using the Microbiome to Unlock the Secrets of Forensic Evidence: Classification of the Body Source of Origin of Human Traces. [(accessed on 20 October 2021)]. Available online: https://www.qiagen.com/us/knowledge-and-support/knowledge-hub/events-and-webinars/webinars/microbiome-to-unlock-the-secrets-of-forensic-evidence.

63. Metcalf J.L., Parfrey L.W., Gonzalez A., Lauber C.L., Knights D., Ackermann G., Humphrey G.C., Gebert M.J., Van Treuren W., Berg-Lyons D., et al. A microbial clock provides an accurate estimate of the postmortem interval in a mouse model system. eLife. 2013;2:e0110. doi: 10.7554/eLife.01104.

64. Inman K., Rudin N. The origin of evidence. Forensic Sci. Int. 2002;126:11–16. doi: 10.1016/S0379-0738(02)00031-2.

65. Bouslimani A., Melnik A.V., Xu Z., Amir A., da Silva R.R., Wang M., Bandeira N., Alexandrov T., Knight R., Dorrestein P.C. Lifestyle chemistries

from phones for individual profiling. Proc. Natl. Acad. Sci. USA. 2016;113:E7645–E7654. doi: 10.1073/pnas.1610019113.
66. Harbison S.A., Fleming R.I. Forensic body fluid identification: State of the art. Res. Rep. Forensic Med. Sci. 2016;6:11–23. doi: 10.2147/RRFMS.S57994.
67. Hanssen E.N., Avershina E., Rudi K., Gill P., Snipen L. Body fluid prediction from microbial patterns for forensic application. Forensic Sci. Int. Genet. 2017;30:10–17. doi: 10.1016/j.fsigen.2017.05.009.
68. Dobay A., Haas C., Fucile G., Downey N., Morrison H.G., Kratzer A., Arora N. Microbiome-based body fluid identification of samples exposed to indoor conditions. Forensic Sci. Int. Genet. 2019;40:105–113. doi: 10.1016/j.fsigen.2019.02.010.
69. Ingold S., Dørum G., Hanson E., Berti A., Branicki W., Brito P., Elsmore P., Gettings K.B., Giangasparo F., Gross T.E., et al. Body fluid identification using a targeted mRNA massively parallel sequencing approach—Results of a EUROFORGEN/EDNAP collaborative exercise. Forensic Sci. Int. Genet. 2018;34:105–115. doi: 10.1016/j.fsigen.2018.01.002.
70. Sauer E., Reinke A.K., Courts C. Differentiation of five body fluids from forensic samples by expression analysis of four microRNAs using quantitative PCR. Forensic Sci. Int. Genet. 2016;22:89–99. doi: 10.1016/j.fsigen.2016.01.018. 11.Hampton-Marcell J., Lopez J.V., Gilbert J.A. The human microbiome: An emerging tool in forensics. Microb. Biotechnol. 2017;10:228–230. doi: 10.1111/1751-7915.12699.
71. Beans C. News feature: Can microbes keep time for forensic investigators? Proc. Natl. Acad. Sci. USA. 2018;115:3–6. doi: 10.1073/pnas.1718156114.

72. Grice E.A., Segre J.A. The skin microbiome. Nat. Rev. Microbiol. 2011;9:244–253. doi: 10.1038/nrmicro2537.
73. Dembinski G.M., Picard C.J. Effects of microbial DNA on human DNA profiles generated using the PowerPlex 16 HS system. J. Forensic Leg. Med. 2017;52:208–214. doi: 10.1016/j.jflm.2017.09.010.
74. Arenas M., Pereira F., Oliveira M., Pinto N., Lopes A.M., Gomes V., Carracedo A., Amorim A. Forensic genetics and genomics: Much more than just a human affair. PLoS Genet. 2017;13:e1006960. doi: 10.1371/journal.pgen.1006960.
75. Kuiper I. Microbial forensics: Next-generation sequencing as catalyst: The use of new sequencing technologies to analyze whole microbial communities could become a powerful tool for forensic and criminal investigations. EMBO Rep. 2016;17:1085–1087. doi: 10.15252/embr.201642794.
76. Leake S.L., Pagni M., Falquet L., Taroni F., Greub G. The salivary microbiome for differentiating individuals: Proof of principle. Microbes Infect. 2016;18:399–405. doi: 10.1016/j.micinf.2016.03.011.
77. Nema V. Microbial Forensics: Beyond a Fascination. In: Dash H., Shrivastava P., Mohapatra B., Das S., editors. DNA Fingerprinting: Advancements and Future Endeavors. Springer; Singapore: 2018. pp. 295–306.
78. Kodama W.A., Xu Z., Metcalf J.L., Song S.J., Harrison N., Knight R., Carter D.O., Happy C.B. Trace Evidence Potential in Postmortem Skin Microbiomes: From Death Scene to Morgue. J. Forensic Sci. 2019;64:791–798. doi: 10.1111/1556-4029.13949.

79. Fierer N., Lauber C.L., Zhou N., McDonald N., Costello E.K., Knight R. Forensic identification using skin bacterial communities. Proc. Natl. Acad. Sci. USA. 2010;107:6477–6481. doi: 10.1073/pnas.1000162107.

80. Schmedes S.E., Sajantila A., Budowle B. Expansion of microbial forensics. J. Clin. Microbiol. 2016;54:1964–1974. doi: 10.1128/JCM.00046-16.

81. Clarke T.H., Gomez A., Singh H., Nelson K.E., Brinkac L.M. Integrating the microbiome as a resource in the forensics toolkit. Forensic Sci. Int. Genet. 2017;30:141–147. doi: 10.1016/j.fsigen.2017.06.008.

82. Budowle B., Connell N.D., Bielecka-Oder A., Colwell R.R., Corbett C.R., Fletcher J., Forsman M., Kadavy D.R., Markotic A., Morse S.A., et al. Validation of high throughput sequencing and microbial forensics applications. Investig. Genet. 2014;5:9. doi: 10.1186/2041-2223-5-9.

83. Giampaoli S., Berti A., Valeriani F., Gianfranceschi G., Piccolella A., Buggiotti L., Rapone C., Valentini A., Ripani L., Spica V.R. Molecular identification of vaginal fluid by microbial signature. Forensic Sci. Int. Genet. 2012;6:559–564. doi: 10.1016/j.fsigen.2012.01.005.

84. Fierer N., Hamady M., Lauber C.L., Knight R. The influence of sex, handedness, and washing on the diversity of hand surface bacteria. Proc. Natl. Acad. Sci. USA. 2008;105:17994–17999. doi: 10.1073/pnas.0807920105.

85. Brinkac L., Clarke T.H., Singh H., Greco C., Gomez A., Torralba M.G., Frank B., Nelson K.E. Spatial and Environmental Variation of the Human Hair Microbiota. Sci. Rep. 2018;8:9017. doi: 10.1038/s41598-018-27100-1.

86. Oh J., Byrd A.L., Park M., NISC Comparative Sequencing Program. Kong H.H., Segre J.A. Temporal Stability of the Human Skin Microbiome. Cell. 2016;165:854–866. doi: 10.1016/j.cell.2016.04.008.

87. Costello E.K., Lauber C.L., Hamady M., Fierer N., Gordon J.I., Knight R. Bacterial Community Variation in Human Body Habitats Across Space and Time. Science. 2009;326:1694–1697. doi: 10.1126/science.1177486.

88. Cullen C.M., Aneja K.K., Beyhan S., Cho C.E., Woloszynek S., Convertino M., McCoy S.J., Zhang Y., Anderson M.Z., Alvarez-Ponce D., et al. Emerging Priorities for Microbiome Research. Front. Microbiol. 2020;11:136. doi: 10.3389/fmicb.2020.00136.

89. Schmedes S.E., Woerner A.E., Budowle B. Forensic human identification using skin microbiomes. Appl. Environ. Microbiol. 2017;83:e01672-17. doi: 10.1128/AEM.01672-17.

90. Schmedes S.E., Woerner A.E., Novroski N.M.M., Wendt F.R., King J.L., Stephens K.M., Budowle B. Targeted sequencing of clade-specific markers from skin microbiomes for forensic human identification. Forensic Sci. Int. Genet. 2018;32:50–61. doi: 10.1016/j.fsigen.2017.10.004.

91. Park J., Kim S.J., Lee J.A., Kim J.W., Kim S.B. Microbial forensic analysis of human-associated bacteria inhabiting hand surface. Forensic Sci. Int. Genet. Suppl. Ser. 2017;6:510–512. doi: 10.1016/j.fsigss.2017.09.210.

92. Flowers L., Grice E.A. The skin microbiota: Balancing risk and reward. Cell Host Microbe. 2020;28:190–200. doi: 10.1016/j.chom.2020.06.017.

93. Edmonds-Wilson S.L., Nurinova N.I., Zapka C.A., Fierer N., Wilson M. Review of human hand microbiome research. J. Dermatol. Sci. 2015;80:3–12. doi: 10.1016/j.jdermsci.2015.07.006.

94. Wilkins D., Leung M.H.Y., Lee P.K.H. Microbiota fingerprints lose individually identifying features over time. Microbiome. 2017;5:1. doi: 10.1186/s40168-016-0209-7.

95. Meadow J.F., Altrichter A.E., Bateman A.C., Stenson J., Brown G.Z., Green J.L., Bohannan B.J.M. Humans differ in their personal microbial cloud. PeerJ. 2015;3:e1258. doi: 10.7717/peerj.1258.
96. Neckovic A., van Oorschot R.A., Szkuta B., Durdle A. Investigation of direct and indirect transfer of microbiomes between individuals. Forensic Sci. Int. Genet. 2020;45:102212. doi: 10.1016/j.fsigen.2019.102212.
97. Hall M.W., Singh N., Ng K.F., Lam D.K., Goldberg M.B., Tenenbaum H.C., Neufeld J.D., Beiko R.G., Senadheera D.B. Inter-personal diversity and temporal dynamics of dental, tongue, and salivary microbiota in the healthy oral cavity. NPJ Biofilms Microbiomes. 2017;3:2. doi: 10.1038/s41522-016-0011-0.
98. Jung J.Y., Yoon H.K., An S., Lee J.W., Ahn E.R., Kim Y.J., Park H.C., Lee K., Hwang J.H., Lim S.K. Rapid oral bacteria detection based on real-time PCR for the forensic identification of saliva. Sci. Rep. 2018;8:10852. doi: 10.1038/s41598-018-29264-2.
99. Miller E.A., Beasley D.E., Dunn R.R., Archie E.A. Lactobacilli Dominance and Vaginal pH: Why Is the Human Vaginal Microbiome Unique? Front. Microbiol. 2016;7:1936. doi: 10.3389/fmicb.2016.01936.
100. Coolen M.J.L., Post E., Davis C.C., Forney J.L. Characterization of Microbial Communities Found in the Human Vagina by Analysis of Terminal Restriction Fragment Length Polymorphisms of 16S rRNA Genes. Appl. Environ. Microbiol. 2005;71:8729–8737. doi: 10.1128/AEM.71.12.8729-8737.2005.
101. Gilbert J., Blaser M.J., Caporaso J.G., Jansson J., Lynch S.V., Knight R. Current understanding of the human microbiome. Nat. Med. 2018;24:392–400. doi: 10.1038/nm.4517.

102. Doi M., Gamo S., Okiura T., Nishimukai H., Asano M. A simple identification method for vaginal secretions using relative quantification of Lactobacillus DNA. Forensic Sci. Int. Genet. 2014;12:93–99. doi: 10.1016/j.fsigen.2014.05.005.

103. López C.D., González D.M., Haas C., Vidaki A., Kayser M. Microbiome-based body site of origin classification of forensically relevant T blood traces. Forensic Sci. Int. Genet. 2020;47:102280. doi: 10.1016/j.fsigen.2020.102280.

104. Tropini C., Earle K.A., Huang K.C., Sonnenburg J.L. The gut microbiome: Connecting spatial organization to function. Cell Host Microbe. 2017;21:433–442. doi: 10.1016/j.chom.2017.03.010.

105. Martínez I., Muller C.E., Walter J. Long-Term Temporal Analysis of the Human Fecal Microbiota Revealed a Stable Core of Dominant Bacterial Species. PLoS ONE. 2013;8:e69621. doi: 10.1371/journal.pone.0069621.

106. Conlon M.A., Bird A.R. The Impact of Diet and Lifestyle on Gut Microbiota and Human Health. Nutrients. 2015;7:17–44. doi: 10.3390/nu7010017.

107. Tridico S.R., Murray D.C., Addison J., Kirkbride K.P., Bunce M. Metagenomic analyses of bacteria on human hairs: A qualitative assessment for applications in forensic science. Investig. Genet. 2014;5:16. doi: 10.1186/s13323-014-0016-5.

108. Williams D.W., Gibson G. Classification of individuals and the potential to detect sexual contact using the microbiome of the pubic region. Forensic Sci. Int. Genet. 2019;41:177–187. doi: 10.1016/j.fsigen.2019.05.004.

109. Molina N.M., Plaza-Diaz J., Vilchez-Vargas R., Sola-Leyva A., Vargas E., Mendoza-Tesarik R., Galán-Lázaro M., de Guevara N.M.-L., Tesarik J., Altmäe S. Assessing the testicular sperm microbiome: A low-biomass site

with abundant contamination. Reprod. Biomed. Online. 2021;43:523–531. doi: 10.1016/j.rbmo.2021.06.021.

110. Farahani L., Tharakan T., Yap T., Ramsay J.W., Jayasena C.N., Minhas S. The semen microbiome and its impact on sperm function and male fertility: A systematic review and meta-analysis. Andrology. 2021;9:115–144. doi: 10.1111/andr.12886.

111. 52.Baud D., Pattaroni C., Vulliemoz N., Castella V., Marsland B.J., Stojanov M. Sperm Microbiota and Its Impact on Semen Parameters. Front. Microbiol. 2019;10:234. doi: 10.3389/fmicb.2019.00234.

112. Quaak F.C.A., van Duijn T., Hoogenboom J., Kloosterman A.D., Kuiper I. Human-associated microbial populations as evidence in forensic casework. Forensic Sci. Int. Genet. 2018;36:176–185. doi: 10.1016/j.fsigen.2018.06.020.

113. Meadow J.F., Altrichter A.E., Green J.L. Mobile phones carry the personal microbiome of their owners. PeerJ. 2014;2:e447. doi: 10.7717/peerj.447.

114. Lax S., Hampton-Marcell J.T., Gibbons S.M., Colares G.B., Smith D., Eisen J.A., Gilbert J.A. Forensic analysis of the microbiome of phones and shoes. Microbiome. 2015;3:21. doi: 10.1186/s40168-015-0082-9.

115. Dong K., Xin Y., Cao F., Huang Z., Sun J., Peng M., Liu W., Shi P. Succession of oral microbiota community as a tool to estimate postmortem interval. Sci. Rep. 2019;9:13063. doi: 10.1038/s41598-019-49338-z.

116. Guo J., Fu X., Liao H., Hu Z., Long L., Yan W., Ding Y., Zha L., Guo Y., Yan J., et al. Potential use of bacterial community succession for estimating post-mortem interval as revealed by high-throughput sequencing. Sci. Rep. 2016;6:24197. doi: 10.1038/srep24197.

117. Cobaugh K.L., Schaeffer S.M., DeBruyn J.M. Functional and Structural Succession of Soil Microbial Communities below Decomposing Human Cadavers. PLoS ONE. 2015;10:e0130201. doi: 10.1371/journal.pone.0130201.
118. Metcalf J.L. Estimating the postmortem interval using microbes: Knowledge gaps and a path to technology adoption. Forensic Sci. Int. Genet. 2019;38:211–218. doi: 10.1016/j.fsigen.2018.11.004.
119. DeBruyn J.M., Hauther K.A. Postmortem succession of gut microbial communities in deceased human subjects. PeerJ. 2017;5:e3437. doi: 10.7717/peerj.3437
120. Belk A., Xu Z.Z., Carter D.O., Lynne A., Bucheli S., Knight R., Metcalf J.L. Microbiome Data Accurately Predicts the Postmortem Interval Using Random Forest Regression Models. Genes. 2018;9:104. doi: 10.3390/genes9020104.
121. Javan G.T., Finley S.J., Abidin Z., Mulle J.G. The Thanatomicrobiome: A Missing Piece of the Microbial Puzzle of Death. Front. Microbiol. 2016;7:225. doi: 10.3389/fmicb.2016.00225.
122. Zhou W., Bian Y. Thanatomicrobiome composition profiling as a tool for forensic investigation. Forensic Sci. Res. 2018;3:105–110. doi: 10.1080/20961790.2018.1466430.
123. Hyde E.R., Haarmann D.P., Lynne A.M., Bucheli S.R., Petrosino J.F. The Living Dead: Bacterial Community Structure of a Cadaver at the Onset and End of the Bloat Stage of Decomposition. PLoS ONE. 2013;8:e77733. doi: 10.1371/journal.pone.0077733.
124. 65.Metcalf J.L., Carter D.O., Knight R. Microbiology of death. Curr. Biol. 2016;26:R561–R563. doi: 10.1016/j.cub.2016.03.042.

125. 66.Handke J., Procopio N., Buckley M., van der Meer D., Williams G., Carr M., Williams A. Successive bacterial colonisation of pork and its implications for forensic investigations. Forensic Sci. Int. 2017;281:1–8. doi: 10.1016/j.forsciint.2017.10.025.
126. Pechal J.L., Schmidt C.J., Jordan H.R., Benbow M.E. A large-scale survey of the postmortem human microbiome, and its potential to provide insight into the living health condition. Sci. Rep. 2018;8:5724. doi: 10.1038/s41598-018-23989-w.
127. Habtom H., Pasternak Z., Matan O., Azulay C., Gafny R., Jurkevitch E. Applying microbial biogeography in soil forensics. Forensic Sci. Int. Genet. 2019;38:195–203. doi: 10.1016/j.fsigen.2018.11.010.
128. Demanèche S., Schauser L., Dawson L., Franqueville L., Simonet P. Microbial soil community analyses for forensic application: Application to a blind test. Forensic Sci. Int. 2017;270:153–158. doi: 10.1016/j.forsciint.2016.12.004.
129. López C.D., Vidaki A., Ralf A., González D.M., Radjabzadeh D., Kraaij R., Uitterlinden A.G., Haas C., Lao O., Kayser M. Novel taxonomy-independent deep learning microbiome approach allows for accurate classification of different forensically relevant human epithelial materials. Forensic Sci. Int. Genet. 2019;41:72–82. doi: 10.1016/j.fsigen.2019.03.015.
130. Williams D.W., Gibson G. Individualization of pubic hair bacterial communities and the effects of storage time and temperature. Forensic Sci. Int. Genet. 2017;26:12–20. doi: 10.1016/j.fsigen.2016.09.006.
131. Song S.J., Amir A., Metcalf J.L., Amato K.R., Xu Z.Z., Humphrey G., Knight R. Preservation methods differ in fecal microbiome stability, affecting suitability for field studies. mSystems. 2016;1:e00021-16. doi:

10.1128/mSystems.00021-16. [DOI] [PMC free article] [PubMed] [Google Scholar]

132. Hanssen E.N., Liland K.H., Gill P., Snipen L. Optimizing body fluid recognition from microbial taxonomic profiles. Forensic Sci. Int. Genet. 2018;37:13–20. doi: 10.1016/j.fsigen.2018.07.012.

133. Grice E.A., Kong H.H., Renaud G., Young A.C., NISC Comparative Sequencing Program. Bouffard G.G., Blakesley R.W., Wolfsberg T.G., Turner M.L., Segre J.A. A diversity profile of the human skin microbiota. Genome Res. 2008;18:1043–1050. doi: 10.1101/gr.075549.107.

134. Flores G.E., Caporaso J.G., Henley J.B., Rideout J.R., Domogala D., Chase J., Leff J.W., Vázquez-Baeza Y., Gonzalez A., Knight R., et al. Temporal variability is a personalized feature of the human microbiome. Genome Biol. 2014;15:531. doi: 10.1186/s13059-014-0531-y.

135. Chase J., Fouquier J., Zare M., Sonderegger D.L., Knight R., Kelley S.T., Siegel J., Caporaso J.G. Geography and location are the primary drivers of office microbiome composition. mSystems. 2016;1:e00022-16. doi: 10.1128/mSystems.00022-16.

136. Tims S., van Wamel W., Endtz H.P., van Belkum A., Kayser M. Microbial DNA fingerprinting of human fingerprints: Dynamic colonization of fingertip microflora challenges human host inferences for forensic purposes. Int. J. Leg. Med. 2010;124:477–481. doi: 10.1007/s00414-009-0352-9.

137. Flores G.E., Bates S.T., Caporaso J.G., Lauber C.L., Leff J.W., Knight R., Fierer N. Diversity, distribution and sources of bacteria in residential kitchens. Environ. Microbiol. 2013;15:588–596. doi: 10.1111/1462-2920.12036.

138. Lax S., Smith D.P., Hampton-Marcell J., Owens S.M., Handley K.M., Scott N.M., Gibbons S.M., Larsen P., Shogan B.D., Weiss S., et al. Longitudinal analysis of microbial interaction between humans and the indoor environment. Science. 2014;345:1048–1052. doi: 10.1126/science.1254529.
139. Song S.J., Lauber C., Costello E.K., Lozupone C.A., Humphrey G., Berg-Lyons D., Caporaso J.G., Knights D., Clemente J.C., Nakielny S., et al. Cohabiting family members share microbiota with one another and with their dogs. eLife. 2013;2:e00458. doi: 10.7554/eLife.00458.
140. Quaak F.C.A., van de Wal Y., Maaskant-van Wijk P.A., Kuiper I. Combining human STR and microbial population profiling: Two case reports. Forensic Sci. Int. Genet. 2018;37:196–199. doi: 10.1016/j.fsigen.2018.08.018.
141. Le Pajolec M.G. French Speaking Working Group of International Society for Forensic Genetics. Personal Communication; Pontoise, France: 2017.
142. Py B., Leonhard J., Martinelle M., Ménabé C. ADN et Justice: L'utilisation de L'empreinte Génétique Dans les Procédures Judiciaires. Presses Universitaires de Nancy—Editions Universitaires de Lorraine; Nancy, France: 2020. Collection «Santé, qualité de vie et handicap».
143. Mégnin, J.-P. *La Faune des cadavres: Application de l'entomologie à la médecine légale*. (Gauthier-Villars et Fils, 1894).
144. Glaister, J. & Brash, J. C. *Medico-legal aspects of the Ruxton case*. (W. Wood & Company, 1937).
145. Lord, W. D., Catts, E. P., Scarboro, D. A. & Hayfield, D. B. The green blowfly, Lucilia illustris, as an indicator of human post-mortem interval: a case of homicide from Fort Lewis, Washington. (Bull. Soc. Vector Ecol., 1986).

146. Introna, F., Campobasso, C. P. & Di Fazio, A. Three case studies in forensic entomology from southern Italy. *J. Forensic Sci.* **43**, 210–214 (1998).
147. Barnes, K. M., Gennard, D. E. & Dixon, R. A. An assessment of the antibacterial activity in larval excretion/secretion of four species of insects recorded in association with corpses, using Lucilia sericata Meigen as the marker species. *Bull. Entomol. Res.* **100**, 635–640 (2010).
148. Zheng, L. *et al.* A survey of bacterial diversity from successive life stages of Black Soldier Fly (Diptera: Stratiomyidae) by using 16S rDNA pyrosequencing. *J. Med. Entomol.* **50**, 647–658 (2013).
149. Singh, B. *et al.* A metagenomic assessment of the bacteria associated with Lucilia sericata and Lucilia cuprina (Diptera: Calliphoridae). *Appl. Microbiol. Biotechnol.* **99**, 869–883 (2015).
150. Tomberlin, J. K. *et al.* A Review of Bacterial Interactions With Blow Flies (Diptera: Calliphoridae) of Medical, Veterinary, and Forensic Importance. *Ann. Entomol. Soc. Am.* **110**, 19–36 (2017).
151. Iancu, L., Junkins, E. N., Necula-Petrareanu, G. & Purcarea, C. Characterizing forensically important insect and microbial community colonization patterns in buried remains. *Sci. Rep.* **8**, 15513 (2018).
152. Ommi, D., Mohammadreza Hashemian, S., Tajbakhsh, E. & Khamesipour, F. Molecular detection and antimicrobial resistance of Aeromonas from houseflies (Musca domestica) in Iran. *Rev. MVZ Córdoba* **20**, 4929–4936 (2015).
153. Waheeda, I. *et al.* Role of housefly (Musca domestica, Diptera; Muscidae) as a disease vector. *J. Entomol. Zool. Stud.* **2**, 159–163 (2014).

154. Solà-Ginés, M. *et al.* Houseflies (Musca domestica) as Vectors for Extended-Spectrum β-Lactamase-Producing Escherichia coli on Spanish Broiler Farms. *Appl. Environ. Microbiol.* **81**, 3604–3611 (2015).

155. Butler, J. F., Garcia-Maruniak, A., Meek, F. & Maruniak, J. E. Wild Florida House Flies (Musca domestica) as Carriers of Pathogenic Bacteria. *Fla. Entomol.* **93**, 218–223 (2010).

156. Royden, A. *et al.* A role for flies (Diptera) in the transmission of Campylobacter to broilers? *Epidemiol. Infect.* **144**, 3326–3334 (2016).

157. Bahrndorff, S., Gill, C., Lowenberger, C., Skovgård, H. & Hald, B. The effects of temperature and innate immunity on transmission of Campylobacter jejuni (Campylobacterales: Campylobacteraceae) between life stages of Musca domestica (Diptera: Muscidae). *J. Med. Entomol.* **51**, 670–677 (2014).

158. Iancu, L., Junkins, E. N. & Purcarea, C. Characterization and microbial analysis of first recorded observation of Conicera similis Haliday (Diptera: Phoridae) in forensic decomposition study in Romania. *J. Forensic Leg. Med.* **58**, 50–55 (2018).

159. Tóth, E. M., Hell, E., Kovács, G., Borsodi, A. K. & Márialigeti, K. Bacteria isolated from the different developmental stages and larval organs of the obligate parasitic fly, Wohlfahrtia magnifica (Diptera: Sarcophagidae). *Microb. Ecol.* **51**, 13–21 (2006).

160. Tóth, E. M. *et al.* Wohlfahrtiimonas chitiniclastica gen. nov., sp. nov., a new gammaproteobacterium isolated from Wohlfahrtia magnifica (Diptera: Sarcophagidae). *Int. J. Syst. Evol. Microbiol.* **58**, 976–981 (2008).

161. Gupta, A. K. *et al.* Ignatzschineria indica sp. nov. and Ignatzschineria ureiclastica sp. nov., isolated from adult flesh flies (Diptera: Sarcophagidae). *Int. J. Syst. Evol. Microbiol.* **61**, 1360–1369 (2011).

162. Cipolla, L. *et al.* Sepsis secondary to complicated skin and soft tissue infection caused by Ignatzschineria indica. First case report in Latin America. *JMM Case Rep.* **5**, e005151 (2018).

163. Katanami, Y. *et al.* Wohlfahrtiimonas chitiniclastica Bacteremia Hospitalized Homeless Man with Squamous Cell Carcinoma. *Emerg. Infect. Dis.* **24**, 1746–1748 (2018).

164. Lysaght, T. B., Wooster, M. E., Jenkins, P. C. & Koniaris, L. G. Myiasis-induced sepsis: a rare case report of Wohlfahrtiimonas chitiniclastica and Ignatzschineria indica bacteremia in the continental United States. *Medicine (Baltimore)* **97**, e13627 (2018).

165. Viero, A., Montisci, M., Pelletti, G. & Vanin, S. Crime scene and body alterations caused by arthropods: implications in death investigation. *Int. J. Legal Med.* **133**, 307–316 (2019).

166. Gupta, A. K. *et al.* Phylogenetic characterization of bacteria in the gut of house flies (Musca domestica L.). *FEMS Microbiol. Ecol.* **79**, 581–593 (2012).

167. Gupta, A. K. *et al.* Molecular phylogenetic profiling of gut-associated bacteria in larvae and adults of flesh flies. *Med. Vet. Entomol.* **28**, 345–354 (2014).

168. Wei, T., Ishida, R., Miyanaga, K. & Tanji, Y. Seasonal variations in bacterial communities and antibiotic-resistant strains associated with green bottle flies (Diptera: Calliphoridae). *Appl. Microbiol. Biotechnol.* **98**, 4197–4208 (2014).

169. Lehrer, A. Z. *Diptera. Familia Calliphoridae. En: Fauna R.S.R. Insecta*. **11** (1972).

170. Kibbe, W. A. OligoCalc: an online oligonucleotide properties calculator. *Nucleic Acids Res.* **35**, W43–46 (2007).

171. Iancu, L., Carter, D. O., Junkins, E. N. & Purcarea, C. Using bacterial and necrophagous insect dynamics for post-mortem interval estimation during cold season: Novel case study in Romania. *Forensic Sci. Int.* **254**, 106–117 (2015).

172. cels.uri.edu/gsc/cndna.html.

173. Smith, K. G. *A manual of forensic entomology*. (Trustees of the British Museum, 1986).

174. Dekeirsschieter, J., Verheggen, F. J., Haubruge, E. & Brostaux, Y. Carrion beetles visiting pig carcasses during early spring in urban, forest and agricultural biotopes of Western. *Europe. J. Insect Sci. Online* **11**, 73 (2011).

175. Catts, E. P. & Haskell, N. H. *Entomology and death: A procedural guide*. (SC Joyce's Print Shop. Clemson, SC., 1990).

176. Metcalf, J. L. *et al.* Microbiome Tools for Forensic Science. *Trends Biotechnol.* **35**, 814–823 (2017).

177. Denno, R. F. & Cothran, W. R. Competitive Interactions and Ecological Strategies of Sarcophagid and Calliphorid Flies Inhabiting Rabbit Carrion. *Ann. Entomol. Soc. Am.* **69**, 109–113 (1976).

178. Byrd, J. H. & Butler, J. F. Effects of temperature on Sarcophaga haemorrhoidalis (Diptera: Sarcophagidae) development. *J. Med. Entomol.* **35**, 694–698 (1998).

179. Gibbs, J. P. & Stanton, E. J. Habitat Fragmentation and Arthropod Community Change: Carrion Beetles, Phoretic Mites, and Flies. *Ecol. Appl.* **11**, 79–85 (2001).
180. Farwig, N., Brandl, R., Siemann, S., Wiener, F. & Müller, J. Decomposition rate of carrion is dependent on composition not abundance of the assemblages of insect scavengers. *Oecologia* **175**, 1291–1300 (2014).
181. Weatherbee, C. R., Pechal, J. L., Stamper, T. & Benbow, M. E. Post-Colonization Interval Estimates Using Multi-Species Calliphoridae Larval Masses and Spatially Distinct Temperature Data Sets: A Case Study. *Insects* **8**, 40 (2017).
182. Zurek, L., Schal, C. & Watson, D. W. Diversity and contribution of the intestinal bacterial community to the development of Musca domestica (Diptera: Muscidae) larvae. *J. Med. Entomol.* **37**, 924–928 (2000).
183. Junqueira, A. C. M. *et al.* The microbiomes of blowflies and houseflies as bacterial transmission reservoirs. *Sci. Rep.* **7** (2017).
184. Scully, E., Friesen, K., Wienhold, B. & Durso, L. M. Microbial Communities Associated With Stable Fly (Diptera: Muscidae) Larvae and Their Developmental Substrates. *Ann. Entomol. Soc. Am.* **110**, 61–72 (2017).
185. Wang, X. *et al.* The gut bacteria across life stages in the synanthropic fly Chrysomya megacephala. *BMC Microbiol.* **18**, 131 (2018).
186. Dharne, M. S. *et al.* Antibacterial activities of multi drug resistant Myroides odoratimimus bacteria isolated from adult flesh flies (Diptera: sarcophagidae) are independent of metallo beta-lactamase gene. *Braz. J. Microbiol.* **39**, 397–404 (2008).
187. Weatherbee, C. R., Pechal, J. L. & Eric Benbow, M. The Dynamic Maggot Mass Microbiome. *Ann. Entomol. Soc. Am.* **110**, 45–53 (2017).

188. Wei, T., Miyanaga, K. & Tanji, Y. Persistence of antibiotic-resistant and -sensitive Proteus mirabilis strains in the digestive tract of the housefly (Musca domestica) and green bottle flies (Calliphoridae). *Appl. Microbiol. Biotechnol.* **98**, 8357–8366 (2014).
189. JD.Wells, L.R.LaMotte, Estimating the postmortem interval J.H. Byrd, J.L. Castner (Eds.), Forensic entomology. The utility of arthropods in legal investigation, CRC Press, Boca Raton , (2001)263-285.
190. M.Coe, The decomposition of elephant carcasses in the Tsavo (East) National Park, Kenya J Arid Environ Res,1(1978) 71-86.
191. K.G.V.Smith, A Manual of Forensic Entomology. British Museum of Natural History, London (1986)207.
192. A.Farinha, CG.Dourado, N.Centeio, AR.Oliveira, D.Dias, MT.Rebelo,. Small bait traps as accurate predictors of dipteran early colonizers in forensic studies. J Insect Sci. 30(2014)14:77. doi: 10.1093/jis/14.1.77.
193. TL.Crippen, B.Singh, Forensic and decomposition microbiology In: Tomberlin JK, Benbow ME, editors. Forensic entomology: international dimensions and frontiers. Boca Raton (FL)p (2015) 249–262.
194. DJ.Wescott , Recent advances in forensic anthropology: decomposition research. Forensic Sci Res. Aug 13;3(4)(2018)327-342. doi: 10.1080/20961790.2018.1488571.
195. MB.Horenstein ,AX.Linhares , Ferradas BRde, Garcia D. Decomposition and dipteran succession in pig carrion in central Argentina: ecological aspects and their importance in forensic science. Med Vet Entomol 24 (2010)16–25. doi: 10.1111/j.1365-2915.2009.00854.x

196. S.Fiedler, K.Kaiser, and B.Fournier,Cadaver imprint on soil chemistry and microbes - Knowns, unknowns, and perspectives. Front.Soil Sci. 3(2023)1107432. doi: 10.3389/fsoil.2023.1107432.

197. R.Janaway, S.Percival, A.Wilson, Decomposition of Human Remains. In: Percival S, Microbiology and Aging: Humana Press. (2009) 313–334.

198. BJ. Jacques, TJ. Bourret, JJ. Shaffer, Role of Fly Cleaning Behavior on Carriage of Escherichia coli and Pseudomonas aeruginosa. J Med Entomol. Nov 7;54(6)(2017)1712-1717. doi: 10.1093/jme/tjx124.

199. V.Balaraman, B.S.Drolet, D.N.Mitzel, W.C. Wilson, J. Owens, N.N. Gaudreault, D.A. Meekins, D. Bold, J.D. Trujillo, L.E. Noronha, et al. Mechanical transmission of SARS-CoV-2 by house flies. Parasites Vectors 14(2021)214.

200. J.-H.Yin, P.J.Kelly, C. Wang, Flies as Vectors and Potential Sentinels for Bacterial Pathogens and Antimicrobial Resistance: A Review. Vet. Sci. 9(2022)300. https:// doi.org/10.3390/vetsci9060300

201. L.Wasala, J.L.Talley, U. DeSilva, J. Fletcher, and A.Wayadande, Transfer of Escherichia coli O157:H7 to spinach by house flies, Musca domestica (Diptera: Muscidae). Phytopathology 103(2013)373-380.

202. R.Fotedar, U.Banerjee, S.J.C.Samantray, Vector potential of hospital houseflies with special reference to Klebsiella species. Epidemiol. Infect. 109(1992)143–147.

203. J.D.Mawak, O.J. Olukose, Vector potential of houseflies (Musca domestica) for pathogenic organisms in Jos, Nigeria. J. Pest Dis. Vector Manag. 7(2006) 418–423.

204. B.Hemmatinezhad, D.Ommi, T.T.Hafshejani, F. Khamesipour, Molecular detection and antimicrobial resistance of Pseudomonas aeruginosa from

houseflies (Musca domestica) in Iran. J. Venom. Anim. Toxins Incl. Trop. Dis. (2015), 21, 18.

205. C.Gill, S. Bahrndorff, C. Lowenberger, Campylobacter jejuni in Musca domestica: An examination of survival and transmission potential in light of the innate immune responses of the house flies. Insect Sci.24 (2017) 584–598 DOI: 10.1111/1744-7917.12353

206. S,Satish, C.Saksham, S.V.Ther,S.Rakesh, S.Ravi,Central Poultry Diagnostic Laboratory (Phoenix Group). Isolation and identification of enterobacterial species from Musca domestica in broiler farms of Madhya Pradesh. Vet. Pract.14(2013) 239–241.

207. B.Greenberg, Flies and Disease. Princeton University.(1971) 447- 452.

208. S.S.Mosallam, "Biological studies of some myiasis producing dipterous flies in Cairo". Ph.D. Thesis, Ain Shams University, Cairo (1980).

209. Norhan E. Salama, Amira Y. Mahfouz, Kotb Hammad, Mohamed M. Kabadaia and Walaa A. Moselhy (2024) Isolation and identification of virulent bacteria from forensic flies as mechanical vectors asso-ciated with a rabbit carcass, *International Journal of Theoretical and Applied Research, 2024, 3,(1): 343-354*

210. N.F.Shaumar, S.K.Mohammed, and S.A.Mohammed, Keys for identification of species of family calliphoridae (Diptera) in Egypt. Journal of the Egyptian Society Parasitology(2)(1989)669-81.

211. T.Whitworth,Keys to the genera and species of blow flies (Diptera: Calliphordae) of America north of Mexico. Proceedings of the Entomological Society of Washington108(3)(2006)689-725. https://www.biodi-versitylibrary.org/part/69166

212. C.J.B.Carvalho ,C.A. and Mello-Patiu, Key to the adults of the most common forensic species of Diptera in South America, Revista Brasileira de Entomologia 53(3)(2008)390–406. https://doi.org/10.1590/S0085-56262008000300012
213. W.C.Rodriguez,W.M. Bass, Insect activity and its relationship to decay rates of human cadavers in East Tennessee. Journal of Forensic Sciences 28(1983)423-432.
214. F.Introna, C.P.Campobasso, M.L.Goff, Entomotoxicology. Forensic Science International 120(2001) 42-47.
215. B.Sabanoglu, O.Sert, Determination of Calliphoridae (Diptera) fauna and seasonal distribution on carrion in Ankara province. Journal of Forensic Sciences 55(4) (2010)1003-1007. DOI: 10.1111/j.1556-4029.2010.01366.x
216. B.Bourel,G.Tournel, V.Hedouin, V.M.Deveaux, M.L.Goff, D.Gosset, Morphine extraction in necrophagous insects remains for determining ante-mortem opiate intoxication. Forensic Science International 120 (2001)127-131.
217. G.M.Mohammed, Zeariya, M.H.Kotb, andM.K. Mohamad, Entomofauna Associated with Certain Animal Carcasses as A human Model in Cairo, Egypt Egypt. Acad. J. Biolog Sci. 10 (2)(2018) 85 – 102 . DOI 10.21608/EAJBSE.2018.38565
218. A.Azwandi, Nina, H.Keterina,L.C. Owen,M.D.Nurizzati, B.Omar, Adult carrion arthropod community in a tropical rainforestof Malaysia: Analysis on three common forensic entomology animal models. Tropical Biomedicine 30(3)(2013)481–494. PMID: 24189678.

219. L.L.M.De Carvalho, and A.X.Linhares, Seasonality of insect succession and pig carcass decomposition in a natural forest area in Southeastern Brazil. Journal of Forensic Science 46 (3)(2001)604–608. PMID: 11372997
220. J.A.Payne, A summer carrion study on the baby pig Sus scrofa L. Ecology 46(1965)592-602.
221. B.D.Turner, Forensic entomology. Forensic Science Progress Vol. 5 (1991)131– 150. Division of Biosphere, London.
222. G.E.Kaiko, T.S.Stappenbeck, Host–microbe interactions shaping the gastrointestinal environment, Trends Immunol 35 (11)(2014) 538–548.DOI 10.1016/j.it.2014.08.002
223. T.L.DeVault,J.O.E. Rhodes, &J.A. Shivik, Scavenging by vertebrates: Behavioral, ecological, and evolutionary perspectives on an important energy transfer pathway in terrestrial ecosystems Oikos 102(2003)225-234.
224. D.W. Hopkins, The role of soil organisms in terrestrial decomposition, Soil Analysis in Forensic Taphonomy, CRC Press, (2008) 61–74. eBook ISBN9780429249495
225. G.M. Mohammed, Zeariya; M.K. Mohamad, Seasonality of Insect Succession and Dog Carcass Decomposition in Different Habitats.Article 3, V. 11(1)(2019) 29-39. DOI 10.21608/EAJBSE.2019.36659
226. B. Suri Babu, K.Rohit, EL-S.Mohamed, S.Mohamed, S.Samy, A.Alaa, A.H.Hassan, M.B.Syed, B.Madhu, Calliphorids as forensic indicator to facilitate PMI estimation: A case study from Chhattisgarh, India. *Journal of King Saud University – Science*, 34, (1) (2022) 101709 DOI:10.1016/j.jksus.2021.101709
227. SP. Donachie, JS., Foster, & MB. Brown, Culture clash: Challenging the dogma of microbial diversity. *The ISME Journal*, 1(2007): 97–102.

228. GP. Fitt, & RW. O'Brien, Bacteria associated with four species of Dacus (Diptera: Tephritidae) and their role in the nutrition of the larvae. *Oecologia*, 67(1985) 447– 454.

229. T.K.Graczyk, R. Knight, R.H.Gilman, and M.R.Cranfield, The role of non-biting flies in the epidemiology of human infectious diseases.Microbes Infect. 3(2001)231-235.

230. E.Arias-Cordero, L.Ping, K.Reichwald, H.Delb, M.Platzer, & W.Boland, Comparative evaluation of the gut microbiota associated with the below- and above-ground life stages (larvae and beetles) of the forest Cockchafer, Melolontha hippocastani. PLoS One 7:(2012) e51557. https://doi.org/10.1371/journal.pone.0051557

231. RT. Jones, LG.Sanchez, & N.Fierer, A cross-taxon analysis of insect associated bacterial diversity. PLoS One 8:(2013) e61218. https://doi.org/10.1371/jour-nal.pone.0061218

232. JH. Yun , S.Woon , R.Tae , W.Whon , M-J et al.Jung , Insect gut bacterial diversity determined by environmental habitat, diet, developmental stage, and phylogeny of host. Applied and Environmental Microbiology 80 (2014) 5254– 5264. DOI: https://doi.org/10.1128/AEM.01226-14

233. F. Amr, M. A. Awad and M. M. Kabadaia: The Insecticidal Activity of Entomopathogenic Bacteria Isolated from *Musca domestica*, *Chrysomya albiceps* and *Lucilia sericata* against the Mosquito Larvae of Culex pipiens, Egypt. Acad. J. Biolog.Sci. (E-Medical Entom. & Parasitology Vol.13(1) (2021)23-28 DOI: 10.21608/E AJBSE.2021.177955.

234. A.N. Mohammed, G.K. Abdel-Latef, N.M. Abdel-Azeem, and K.M.El-Dakhly, Ecological study on antimicrobial-resistant zoonotic bacteria

transmitted by flies in cattle farms. *Parasitology research*, 31(2016) 1-8. DOI: 10.1007/s00436-016-5154-7

235. M.Cheesbrough, District Laboratory Practice in Tropical Countries, Cambridge University Press, Cambridge, UK, 2nd edition, (2006).
236. A.Behar, E.Jurkevitch, B.YUVAL, a. Bringing back the fruit into fruit fly-bacteria interactions. Mol Ecol 17(2008)1375–1386.
237. N.Thaochan, A.Chinajariyawong, Attraction of Bactrocera cucurbitae and B. papayae (Diptera: Tephritidae) to the odor of the bacterium Enterobacter cloacae. Philipp Agric Scientist 94 (2011) 83–87.
238. M.Förster, S.Klimpel, H. Mehlhorn, K.Sievert,S. Messler, and K.Pfeffer, Pilot study on synanthropic flies (eg Musca, Sarcophaga, Calliphora, Fannia, Lucilia, and Stomoxys) as vectors of pathogenic microorganisms. Parasitology research,101(1)(2007) 243-246. DOI: 10.1007/s00436-007-0522-y
239. W.A.Nazmi,B.Seleena,H.L. Lee, J.Jeffery, T.A.R.Rogayah, and M.A.Sofian, Bacteria fauna from the house fly, Musca domestica (L.). Trop Biomed, 22(2)(2005) 225-231. PMID: 16883292
240. J.F.Butler, A.Garcia-Maruniak, F. Meek, and J.E.Maruniak, Wild Florida house flies (Musca domestica) domestica) as carriers of pathogenic bacteria.Florida Entomologist, 93(2)(2010) 218-223. DOI:10.1653/024.093.0211
241. L.C. Choo, A.A. Saleha, S.S. Wai, and N. Fauziah, Isolation of *Campylobacter* and *Salmonella* from houseflies (*Musca domestica*) in a university campus and a poultry farm in Selangor, Malaysia. Tropical biomedicine, 28 (1) (2011) 16-20. PMID: 21602764.

242. T. Chaiwong, T. Srivoramas, K. Sukontason, M.R. Sanford, andK.L. Sukontason, Bacterial fauna associated with the blow fly, *Chrysomya megacephala* (F.) in U bon Ratchathani Province of Northeast Thailand. International Journal of Parasitology Research, 4(1) (2012) 71. DOI:10.9735/0975-3702.4.1.71-74
243. M.A. Habeeb, and M.A. Mahdi: Mechanical transmission of bacteria via animal agent's true fly species. Advanced Studies in Biology, 4(12) (2012) 583-591. DOI: http://dx.doi.org/10.9735/0975-3702.4.1.71-74
244. A.S. Ahmed, K. M. Ahmed, S. S. and Salih, Isolation and Identification of Bacterial Isolates from House Flies in Sulaymaniya City. *Eng. &Tech. Journal*, 31 (1) (2013) 24-33. DOI 10.30684/etj.31.1B.4
245. M.H. Motazedian, D. Mehrabani, and G. Mehrabani, The Role of Musca domestica as a Carrier of Parasites in Shiraz, Southern Iran. Academic *Journal of Entomology*, 7 (3) (2014) 84-87. DOI:10.5829/idosi.aje.2014.7.3.83158
246. M. Davies, Isolation and characterisation of bacteria associated with flying insects in hospitals, with particular emphasis on *Clostridium difficile*, PhD thesis, Aston University(2015), 285.
247. Kamaluddin, M., Shariff, N. & Matsaat, G. Mechanical profiles of murder and murderers: An extensive review. *Malays. J. Pathol.* **40**, 10 (2018).
248. Junkins, E. N. & Carter, D. O. Relationships between Human Remains, Graves and the Depositional Environment. In *Taphonomy of Human Remains: Forensic Analysis of the Dead and the Depositional Environment* (eds Schotsmans, E. M. J., Mrquez-Grant, N.& Forbes, S. L.) 143–154, https://doi.org/10.1002/9781118953358.ch11 (John Wiley & Sons, Ltd, 2017).

249. Bergeret, L.F. *Infanticide, momification naturelle du cadavre*. (Arbois: impr. de E. Javel, 1864).
250. Smith, K. G. *A manual of forensic entomology*. (Trustees of the British Museum, 1986).
251. Anderson, G. S. Determining time of death using blow fly eggs in the early postmortem interval. *Int. J. Legal Med.* **118** (2004).
252. Anderson, G. S. Comparison of decomposition rates and faunal colonization of carrion in indoor and outdoor environments:decomposition rates and faunal colonization of carrion. *J. Forensic Sci.* **56**, 136–142 (2011).
253. Bharti, M. & Singh, D. Insect Faunal Succession on Decaying Rabbit Carcasses in Punjab, India. *J. Forensic Sci.* **48**, 2001358 (2003).
254. Carter, D. O., Yellowlees, D. & Tibbett, M. Cadaver decomposition in terrestrial ecosystems. *Naturwissenschaften* **94**, 12–24 (2006).
255. Benbow, M. E., Lewis, A. J., Tomberlin, J. K. & Pechal, J. L. Seasonal Necrophagous Insect Community Assembly During VertebrateCarrion Decomposition. *J. Med. Entomol.* **50**, 440–450 (2013).
256. Finley, S. J., Benbow, M. E. & Javan, G. T. Microbial communities associated with human decomposition and their potential use aspostmortem clocks. *Int. J. Legal Med.* **129**, 623–632 (2015).
257. Metcalf, J. L. *et al.* Microbial community assembly and metabolic function during mammalian corpse decomposition. *Science* 351,158–162 (2016).
258. Carter, D. O. & Tibbett, M. Does repeated burial of skeletal muscle tissue (Ovis aries) in soil affect subsequent decomposition? *Appl. Soil Ecol.* 40, 529–535 (2008).
259. Gunn, A. & Bird, J. The ability of the blowflies *Calliphora vomitoria* (Linnaeus), *Calliphora vicina* (Rob-Desvoidy) and Luciliasericata (Meigen)

(Diptera: Calliphoridae) and the muscid flies *Muscina stabulans* (Fallén) and *Muscina prolapsa* (Harris) (Diptera: Muscidae) to colonise buried remains. *Forensic Sci. Int.* 207, 198–204 (2011).

260. Wei, T., Miyanaga, K. & Tanji, Y. Persistence of antibiotic-resistant and -sensitive *Proteus mirabilis* strains in the digestive tract of the housefly (Musca domestica) and green bottle flies (Calliphoridae). *Appl. Microbiol. Biotechnol.* 98, 8357–8366 (2014).

261. Gunn, A. The colonisation of remains by the muscid flies *Muscina stabulans* (Fallén) and Muscina prolapsa (Harris) (Diptera: Muscidae). *Forensic Sci. Int.* 266, 349–356 (2016).

262. Janaway, R. The preservation of organic materials in association with metal artefacts deposited in inhumation graves. In *Death,decay and reconstruction: approaches to archaeology and forensic science* (eds Boddington, A., Garland, A. & Janaway, R.) 127–141(Manchester University Press, 1987).

263. Janaway, R. The decay of buried human remains and their associated materials. In *Studies in crime: an introduction to forensic archaeology* (eds Hunter, J., Roberts, C. & Martin, A.) 58–85 (Routledge, 1996).

264. Janaway, R. C., Percival, S. L. & Wilson, A. S. Decomposition of Human Remains. In *Microbiology and Aging* (ed. Percival, S. L.)313–334, https://doi.org/10.1007/978-1-59745-327-1_14 (Humana Press, 2009).

265. Szpila, K., Voss, J. G. & Pape, T. A new dipteran forensic indicator in buried bodies. *Med. Vet. Entomol.* https://doi.org/10.1111/j.1365-2915.2010.00883.x (2010).

266. Carter, D. O., Yellowlees, D. & Tibbett, M. Moisture can be the dominant environmental parameter governing cadaver decomposition in soil. *Forensic Sci. Int.* 200, 60–66 (2010).

267. Mariani, R., Garca-Mancuso, R., Varela, G. L. & Inda, A. M. Entomofauna of a buried body: Study of the exhumation of a humancadaver in Buenos Aires, Argentina. *Forensic Sci. Int.* 237, 19–26 (2014).
268. Motter, M. G. A Contribution to the Study of the Fauna of the Grave. A Study of on Hundred and Fifty Disinterments, with Some Additional Experimental Observations. *J. N. Y. Entomol. Soc.* **6**, 201–231 (1898).
269. Lord, W. D., Adkins, T. R. & Catts, E. P. Use of *Synthesiomyia nudesita* (Van Der Wulp) (Diptera: Muscidae) and *Calliphora vicina* (Robineau-Desvoidy) (Diptera: Calliphoridae) to estimate the time of death of a body buried under a house. *J. Agric. Entomol.* (1992).
270. Rodriguez, W. C. & Bass, W. M. Decomposition of buried bodies and methods that may aid in their location. *J. Forensic Sci.* **30**,836–852 (1985).
271. Rysavy, N. M. & Goff, M. L. Preliminary Observations of Arthropods Associated with Buried Carrion on Oahu. *J. Forensic Sci.* **60**,462–467 (2015).
272. Finley, S. J., Pechal, J. L., Benbow, M. E., Robertson, B. K. & Javan, G. T. Microbial Signatures of Cadaver Gravesoil DuringDecomposition. *Microb. Ecol.* **71**, 524–529 (2016).
273. VanLaerhoven, S. L. & Anderson, G. S. Insect succession on buried carrion in two biogeoclimatic zones of British Columbia. *J.Forensic Sci.* **44**, 32–43 (1999).
274. Lowe, A. C. *et al.* The effect of soil texture on the degradation of textiles associated with buried bodies. *Forensic Sci. Int.* **231**,331–339 (2013).
275. Bernhardt, V. *et al.* Muscina prolapsa (Harris 1780): Ein bislang unterschütztes Werkzeug der forensischen Entomologie.*Rechtsmedizin* **26**, 97–102 (2016).

276. Marais-Werner, A., Myburgh, J., Meyer, A., Nienaber, W. & Steyn, M. Decomposition patterns of buried remains at differentintervals in the Central Highveld region of South Africa. *Med. Sci. Law* **57**, 115–123 (2017).
277. Gaudry, E. The Insects Colonisation of Buried Remains. In *Current Concepts in Forensic Entomology* (eds Amendt, J., Goff, M. L.,Campobasso, C. P. & Grassberger, M.) 273–311, https://doi.org/10.1007/978-1-4020-9684-6_13 (Springer Netherlands, 2010).
278. Pechal, J. L. *et al.* Microbial Community Functional Change during Vertebrate Carrion Decomposition. *PLoS ONE* 8, e79035(2013).
279. Finley, S. J., Benbow, M. E. & Javan, G. T. Potential applications of soil microbial ecology and next-generation sequencing incriminal investigations. *Appl. Soil Ecol.* 88, 69–78 (2015).
280. Goff, M. L. Early Postmortem Changes and Stages of Decomposition. In *Current Concepts in Forensic Entomology* (eds Amendt, J.,Goff, M. L., Campobasso, C. P. & Grassberger, M.) 1–24, https://doi.org/10.1007/978-1-4020-9684-6_1 (Springer Netherlands,2009).
281. Wilson, A. S. *et al.* Modelling the buried human body environment in upland climes using three contrasting field sites. *Forensic Sci.Int.* 169, 6–18 (2007).
282. Haglund, W. D. & Sorg, M. H. *Forensic taphonomy: the postmortem fate of human remains*. (CRC Press, 1997).
283. Forbes, S. L. Potential determinants of postmortem and post burial interval of buried remains. In *Soil analysis in forensic taphonomy* (eds Tibbett, M. & Carter, D. O.) 225–246 (CRC Press, 2008).
284. Payne, J. A., King, E. W. & Beinhart, G. Arthropod Succession and Decomposition of Buried Pigs. *Nature* 219, 1180–1181 (1968).

285. Rodriguez, W. C. & Bass, W. M. Insect Activity and its Relationship to Decay Rates of Human Cadavers in East Tennessee. *J. Forensic Sci.* 28, 11524J (1983).
286. Bourel, B., Tournel, G., Hedouin, V. & Gosset, D. Entomofauna of buried bodies in northern France. *Int. J. Legal Med.* 118 (2004).
287. Pechal, J. L. *et al.* The potential use of bacterial community succession in forensics as described by high throughput metagenomicsequencing. *Int. J. Legal Med.* 128, 193–205 (2014).
288. Hyde, E. R., Haarmann, D. P., Lynne, A. M., Bucheli, S. R. & Petrosino, J. F. The Living Dead: Bacterial Community Structure of aCadaver at the Onset and End of the Bloat Stage of Decomposition. *PLoS ONE* 8, e77733 (2013).
289. Hyde, E. R., Haarmann, D. P., Petrosino, J. F., Lynne, A. M. & Bucheli, S. R. Initial insights into bacterial succession during humandecomposition. *Int. J. Legal Med.* 129, 661–671 (2015).
290. Carter, D. O., Metcalf, J. L., Bibat, A. & Knight, R. Seasonal variation of postmortem microbial communities. *Forensic Sci. Med.Pathol.* 11, 202–207 (2015).
291. Javan, G. T., Finley, S. J., Abidin, Z. & Mulle, J. G. The Thanatomicrobiome: A Missing Piece of the Microbial Puzzle of Death. *Front.Microbiol.* 7 (2016).
292. Guo, J. *et al.* Potential use of bacterial community succession for estimating post-mortem interval as revealed by high-throughputsequencing. *Sci. Rep.* 6 (2016).

293. Chimutsa, M., Olakanye, A. O., Thompson, T. J. U. & Ralebitso-Senior, T. K. Soil fungal community shift evaluation as a potential cadaver decomposition indicator. *Forensic Sci. Int.* 257, 155–159 (2015).
294. Cobaugh, K. L., Schaeffer, S. M. & DeBruyn, J. M. Functional and Structural Succession of Soil Microbial Communities belowDecomposing Human Cadavers. *PLOS ONE* 10, e0130201 (2015)
295. Metcalf, J. L. *et al.* A microbial clock provides an accurate estimate of the postmortem interval in a mouse model system. *eLife* 2(2013).
296. Weatherbee, C. R., Pechal, J. L., Stamper, T. & Benbow, M. E. Post-Colonization Interval Estimates Using Multi-SpeciesCalliphoridae Larval Masses and Spatially Distinct Temperature Data Sets: A Case Study. *Insects* 8, 40 (2017).
297. Hauther, K. A., Cobaugh, K. L., Jantz, L. M., Sparer, T. E. & DeBruyn, J. M. Estimating Time Since Death from Postmortem HumanGut Microbial Communities. *J. Forensic Sci.* 60, 1234–1240 (2015).
298. Santo Domingo, J. W., Siefring, S. C. & Haugland, R. A. Real-time PCR method to detect Enterococcus faecalis in water. *Biotechnol. Lett.* 25, 261–265 (2003).
299. Guo, X. *et al.* Development of a real-time PCR method for Firmicutes and Bacteroidetes in faeces and its application to quantify intestinal population of obese and lean pigs. *Lett. Appl. Microbiol.* 47, 367–373 (2008).
300. Hermann-Bank, M., Skovgaard, K., Stockmarr, A., Larsen, N. & Mőlbak, L. The Gut Microbiotassay: a high-throughput qPCR approach combinable with next generation sequencing to study gut microbial diversity. *BMC Genomics* 14, 788 (2013).

301. Veskoukis, A. S. *et al.* Effects of xanthine oxidase inhibition on oxidative stress and swimming performance in rats. *Appl. Physiol. Nutr. Metab. Physiol. Appl. Nutr. Metab.* 33, 1140–1154 (2008).

302. Booth, F. W. & Laye, M. J. Lack of adequate appreciation of physical exercise's complexities can pre-empt appropriate design and interpretation in scientific discovery. *J. Physiol.* 587, 5527–5539 (2009).

303. Nikolaidis, M. G. *et al.* Effect of chronic wheel running on the fatty acid composition of phospholipids and triacylglycerols in rat serum, skeletal muscle and heart. *Acta Physiol. Scand.* 181, 199–208 (2004).

304. Allen, D. G., Lamb, G. D. & Westerblad, H. Skeletal muscle fatigue: cellular mechanisms. *Physiol. Rev.* 88, 287–332 (2008).

305. Kyparos, A., Feeback, D. L., Layne, C. S., Martinez, D. A. & Clarke, M. S. F. Mechanical stimulation of the plantar foot surface attenuates soleus muscle atrophy induced by hindlimb unloading in rats. *J. Appl. Physiol. Bethesda Md 1985* 99, 739–746 (2005).

306. R҉ckl, K. S. C., Witczak, C. A. & Goodyear, L. J. Signaling mechanisms in skeletal muscle: acute responses and chronic adaptations to exercise. *IUBMB Life* 60, 145–153 (2008).

307. Carter, D. O., Yellowlees, D. & Tibbett, M. Temperature affects microbial decomposition of cadavers (Rattus rattus) in contrasting soils. *Appl. Soil Ecol.* 40, 129–137 (2008).

308. Loveland, P. A Handbook of Soil Terminology, Correlation andClassification - edited by Krasilnikov, Pavel, IbٽIez Martي, Juan- Jose, Arnold, Richard & Shoba, Serghei. *Eur. J. Soil Sci.* 61, 316–317 (2010).

309. Goutianos, G. *et al.* The rat adequately reflects human responses to exercise in blood biochemical profile: a comparative study. *Physiol. Rep.* 3, e12293 (2015).

310. Meteo Romania | Romanian national administration wheater service site. Available at: http://www.meteoromania.ro/anm2/. (Accessed: 1st March 2016).

311. Disney, R. H. L. *Scuttle flies: Diptera, Phoridae (except Megaselia).* 6, (Royal Entomological Society of London, 1983).

312. Gregor, F. *The Muscidae (Diptera) of Central Europe.* (Masaryk Univ., 2002).

313. Grzywacz, A., Hall, M. J. R. & Pape, T. Morphology successfully separates third instar larvae of *Muscina*: Identification of third instars of Muscina. *Med. Vet. Entomol.* 29, 314–329 (2015).

314. Hebert, P. D. N., Cywinska, A., Ball, S. L. & deWaard, J. R. Biological identifications through DNA barcodes. *Proc. Biol. Sci.* 270,313–321 (2003).

315. Folmer, O., Black, M., Hoeh, W., Lutz, R. & Vrijenhoek, R. DNA primers for amplification of mitochondrial cytochrome c oxidasesubunit I from diverse metazoan invertebrates. *Mol. Mar. Biol. Biotechnol.* 3, 294–299 (1994).

316. National Center for Biotechnology Information. Available at: https://www.ncbi.nlm.nih.gov/. (Accessed: 15th March 2017).

317. Sequence Assembly and Alignment Software - CodonCode. Available at: http://www.codoncode.com/. (Accessed: 26th April 2017).

318. Takahashi, S., Tomita, J., Nishioka, K., Hisada, T. & Nishijima, M. Development of a Prokaryotic Universal Primer for SimultaneousAnalysis of

Bacteria and Archaea Using Next-Generation Sequencing. *PLoS ONE* 9, e105592 (2014).

319. Zhang, J., Kobert, K., Flouri, T. & Stamatakis, A. PEAR: a fast and accurate Illumina Paired-End reAd mergeR. *Bioinformatics* 30,614–620 (2014).

320. Edgar, R. C. UPARSE: highly accurate OTU sequences from microbial amplicon reads. *Nat. Methods* 10, 996–998 (2013).

321. Caporaso, J. G. *et al.* QIIME allows analysis of high-throughput community sequencing data. *Nat. Methods* 7, 335–336 (2010).

322. Quast, C. *et al.* The SILVA ribosomal RNA gene database project: improved data processing and web-based tools. *Nucleic Acids Res.*41, D590–D596 (2012).

323. Iancu, L., Junkins, E. N. & Purcarea, C. Characterization and microbial analysis of first recorded observation of Conicera similisHaliday (Diptera: Phoridae) in forensic decomposition study in Romania. *J. Forensic Leg. Med.* 58, 50–55 (2018).

324. Tonooka, T. *et al.* Detection and Quantification of Four Species of the Genus *Clostridium* in Infant Feces. *Microbiol. Immunol.* 49,987–992 (2005).

325. Clifford, R. J. *et al.* Detection of Bacterial 16S rRNA and Identification of Four Clinically Important Bacteria by Real-Time PCR.*PLoS ONE* **7**, e48558 (2012).

326. Hammer, O., Harper, A. T. D. & Ryan, D. P. PAST: Paleontological Statistics Software Package for Education and Data Analysis.*Palaeontol. Electron.* 4, 4–9 (2001).

327. Forbes, S. L., Perrault, K. A. & Comstock, J. L. Microscopic Post-Mortem Changes: the Chemistry of Decomposition. In *Taphonomyof Human Remains: Forensic Analysis of the Dead and the* Depositional *Environment*

(eds Schotsmans, E. M. J., Marquez-Grant, N.& Forbes, S. L.) 26–38, https://doi.org/10.1002/9781118953358.ch2 (John Wiley & Sons, Ltd, 2017).
328. Stuart, B. H. & Ueland, M. Degradation of Clothing in Depositional Environments. In *Taphonomy of Human Remains: ForensicAnalysis of the Dead and the* Depositional *Environment* (eds Schotsmans, E. M. J., Marquez-Grant, N. & Forbes, S. L.) 120–133,https://doi.org/10.1002/9781118953358.ch9 (John Wiley & Sons, Ltd, 2017).
329. Pounder, D. Postmortem interval. In *Encyclopaedia of* Forensic *Sciences* (eds Siegel, J., Knupfer, G. & Saukko, P.) 1167–1172(Academic Press, 2000).
330. Gennard, D. E. *Forensic entomology: an introduction*. (John Wiley & Sons, 2007).
331. Rodriguez, W. C. 3rd. Decomposition of buried and submerged bodies. In *Forensic taphonomy. The postmortem fate of human remains* (eds Haglund, W. D. & Sorg, M. H.) (CRC Press, 1997).
332. Pastula, E. C. & Merritt, R. W. Insect arrival pattern and succession on buried carrion in Michigan. *J. Med. Entomol.* 50, 432–439(2013).
333. Turner, B. & Wiltshire, P. Experimental validation of forensic evidence: a study of the decomposition of buried pigs in a heavy claysoil. *Forensic Sci. Int.* 101, 113–122 (1999).
334. Vanin, S. & Huchet, J.-B. Forensic Entomology and Funerary Archaeoentomology. In *Taphonomy of Human Remains: ForensicAnalysis of the Dead and the Depositional Environment* (eds Schotsmans, E. M. J., MJrquez-Grant, N. & Forbes, S. L.) 167–186,

https://doi.org/10.1002/9781118953358.ch13 (John Wiley & Sons, Ltd, 2017).
335. Schroeder, H., Klotzbach, H. & Püschel, K. Insects' colonization of human corpses in warm and cold season. *Leg. Med.* 5, S372–S374 (2003).
336. Skidmore, P. *The biology of the Muscidae of the world*. (Springer, 1985).
337. Disney, R. H. L. *Scuttle Flies: The Phoridae*. https://doi.org/10.1007/978-94-011-1288-8 (Springer, 1994).
338. Leclercq, M. Entomologie et médecine légale: importance des Phorides sur les cadavres humains. In *Annales de la SociétéEntomologique de France* 566–568 (1999).
339. Mégnin, J.-P. *La Faune des cadavres: Application de l'entomologie à la médecine légale*. (Gauthier-Villars et Fils, 1894).
340. Lundt, H. Kologische Untersuchungen über die tierische Besiedlung von Aas im Boden. *Pedobiologia* 4, 158–180 (1964).
341. Anderson, G. S. Wildlife Forensic Entomology: Determining Time of Death in Two Illegally Killed Black Bear Cubs. *J. Forensic Sci.*44, 14567J (1999).
342. Gaudry, E. *et al.* Burial of lamb carcasses at 3 different depths: impact on the colonization by necrophagous insects. *Proc. FourthMeet. Eur. Assoc. Forensic Entomol. Bari Italy* (2006).
343. Singh, B. *et al.* A metagenomic assessment of the bacteria associated with *Lucilia sericata* and *Lucilia cuprina* (Diptera: Calliphoridae). *Appl. Microbiol. Biotechnol.* 99, 869–883 (2015).
344. Zheng, L. *et al.* A survey of bacterial diversity from successive life stages of Black Soldier Fly (Diptera: Stratiomyidae) by using 16SrDNA pyrosequencing. *J. Med. Entomol.* 50, 647–658 (2013).

345. Damann, F. E. Bacterial Symbionts and Taphonomic Agents of Humans. In *Taphonomy of Human Remains: Forensic Analysis of theDead and the Depositional Environment* (eds Schotsmans, E. M. J., MUrquez-Grant, N. & Forbes, S. L.) 155–166, https://doi.org/10.1002/9781118953358.ch12 (John Wiley & Sons, Ltd, 2017).
346. Metcalf, J. L. *et al.* Microbiome Tools for Forensic Science. *Trends Biotechnol.* 35, 814–823 (2017).
347. DeBruyn, J. M. & Hauther, K. A. Postmortem succession of gut microbial communities in deceased human subjects. *PeerJ* **5**, e3437(2017).
348. Li, D. *et al.* Microbial Biogeography and Core Microbiota of the Rat Digestive Tract. *Sci. Rep.* 8, 45840 (2017).
349. Arumugam, M. *et al.* Enterotypes of the human gut microbiome. *Nature* 473, 174–180 (2011).
350. Ventura, M. *et al.* Genomics of Actinobacteria: Tracing the Evolutionary History of an Ancient Phylum. *Microbiol. Mol. Biol. Rev.*71, 495–548 (2007).
351. Nishida, A. H. & Ochman, H. Rates of gut microbiome divergence in mammals. *Mol. Ecol.* **27**, 1884–1897 (2018).
352. Berg, R. The indigenous gastrointestinal microflora. *Trends Microbiol.* 4, 430–435 (1996).
353. Ryan, K. J. & Ray, C. G. *Sherris Medical Microbiology*. (McGraw Hill Professional, 2003).
354. Huycke, M. M., Spiegel, C. A. & Gilmore, M. S. Bacteremia caused by hemolytic, high-level gentamicin-resistant *Enterococcus faecalis*. *Antimicrob. Agents Chemother.* 35, 1626–1634 (1991).

355. Rocas, I., Siqueirajr, J. & Santos, K. Association of *Enterococcus faecalis* with different forms of periradicular diseases. *J. Endod.* 30, 315–320 (2004).
356. Murray, B. Diversity among Multidrug-Resistant Enterococci. *Emerg. Infect. Dis.* 4, 37–47 (1998).
357. Stuart, C., Schwartz, S., Beeson, T. & Owatz, C. *Enterococcus faecalis*: its role in root canal treatment failure and current conceptsin retreatment. *J. Endod.* 32, 93–98 (2006).
358. de la Maza, L. M. *Colour Atlas of Medical Bacteriology*. 1, (ASM Press, 2004).
359. Holt, K. & Sneath, S. W. *Bergey's Manual of determinative bacteriology* (1994).
360. Sekirov, I., Russell, S. L., Antunes, L. C. M. & Finlay, B. B. Gut Microbiota in Health and Disease. *Physiol. Rev.* 90, 859–904 (2010).
361. Shinha, T. & Hadi, C. *Clostridium paraputrificum* Bacteremia Associated with Colonic Necrosis in a Patient withAIDS. *Case Rep.Infect. Dis.* **2015**, 1–3 (2015).
362. Evvyernie, D. *et al.* Identification and characterization of *Clostridium paraputrificum* M-21, a chitinolytic, mesophilic and hydrogen-producing bacterium. *J. Biosci. Bioeng.* 89, 596–601 (2000).
363. Kiu, R. *et al.* Preterm infant-associated *Clostridium tertium*, *Clostridium cadaveris*, and *Clostridium paraputrificum* strains: genomic and evolutionary insights. *Genome Biol. Evol.* 9, 2707–2714 (2017).
364. Anderson, G. S. and Sherah L. Van Laerhoven (1996). Initial studies on insect succession on carrion in south western British Columbia. *J. Forensic Sci.* 41: 617-625.

365. Marchenko, M. I. (1988). Medico-legal relevance of corpse entomofauna for the determination of the time since death. *Acta Med. Leg. Soc.* (Liege) 38: 257-302.
366. Catts, E. P., and M. L. Goff. (1992). Forensic entomology in criminal investigations. *Annu. Rev. Entomol.* 37: 253-272.
367. Anderson, G. S. (1997). The use of insects to determine time of decapitation: a case-study from British Columbia. J. Forensic Sci. 42: 947-950.
368. Amendt, J., R. Krettek, and R. Zehner. (2004). Forensic Entomology. Naturwissenschaften 91: 51-65.
369. Campobasso, C. P., J. G. Linville, J. D. Wells, and F. Introna. (2005). Forensic genetic analysis of insect gut contents. *Am. J. Forensic Med.Pathol.* 26: 161-165
370. Gomes, L., W. A. Godoy, and C. J. Von Zuben (2006). A review of postfeeding larval dispersal in blowflies: implications for forensic entomology. Naturwissenschaften 93: 207-215.
371. Kashyap, V. K., and V. V. Pillay. (1989). Efficacy of entomological method in estimation of postmortem interval: a comparative analysis. *Forensic Sci. Int.* 40: 245-250.
372. Amendt, J., C. P. Campobasso, E. Gaudry, C. Reiter, H. N. LeBlanc, and M. J. Hall. (2007) European Association for Forensic Entomology. Best practice in forensic entomology--standards and guidelines. *Int. J. Legal Med.* 121: 90-104.
373. Erzinçlioglu, Z. (2003). Forensic entomology. *Clin. Med.* 3: 74-76.
374. Benecke, M. and J. D. Wells (2001). DNA techniques for forensic entomology. Forensic entomology: Utility of arthropods in legal investigations. CRC Press, Boca Raton: 341-352.

375. Campobasso, C. P., and F. Introna (2001). The forensic entomologist in the context of the forensic pathologist's role. *Forensic Sci. Int.* 120: 132-139.

376. Edirisinghe, J. S., and J. P. Edirisinghe. (1994). Forensic entomology. *Ceylon Med.J.* 39: 121-123

377. Otranto, D., and J. R. Stevens. (2002). Molecular approaches to the study of myiasis-causing larvae. *Int. J. Parasitol.* 32: 1345-1360.

378. Jean-Baptiste Baillière (1855). Infanticide, Momification naturelle du cadavr', Annalesd' hygiene publique et de médecinelégale, série 2, no 4.-Paris.

379. Leclercq M and Valliant F. (1992). Entomologie Et Medicine Legale: Une Observation Inedited. *Annals Society Entomology France*; 28 (1): 3-8.

380. Joseph I, Mathew DG, Sathyan P, Vargheese G. (2011). The use of insects in forensic investigations: An overview on the scope of forensic entomology. *J Forensic Dent Sci.*;3(2):89-91.

381. LeBlanc HN, Logan JG. (2010). Exploiting Insect Olfaction in Forensic Entomology. In: Amendt J, Goff ML, Campobasso CP, Grassberger M (eds). Current Concepts in Forensic Entomology. Springer, Netherlands.;205-221.

382. Tullis K, Goff ML. (1987). Arthropod succession in exposed carrion in atropical rainforest on O 'ahu Island, Hawai. *J Med Entomol.*;24:332-339.

383. Beyer J C, Enos W F and Stajic M (1980). Drug identification through analysis of maggots. Journal of Forensic Science. 25: 411-412.

384. Goff ML. (2000). A Fly for The Prosecution: How Insect Evidence Helps Solve Crimes. Harvard University Press, Cambridge. 2nd ed.; p.1-225

385. Goff ML, Omori AI and Goodbrod JR (1989). Effect of Cocaine in Tissues on the Development Rate of *Boettohersca peregrina* (Diptera: Sarcophagidae). *Journal of Medical Entomology*, 26(2): 91-93.

386. Kintz P, Tracqui A, Ludes B, Waller J, Bonkhabza A, Mangin P, Lugnier AA and Chaumont AJ. (1990). Fly Larvae and Their Relevance in Forensic Toxicology. *American Journal of Forensic Medicine and Pathology*, 11 (1): 63-65.

387. Kintz P, Tracqui A and Mangin P. (1990). Toxicology and Fly Larvae on a Putrefied Corpse. *Journal of Forensic Science Society*, (4): 243-246.

388. Goff ML, Brown WA and Omori AI.(1992). Preliminary Observations of the Effect of Methamphetamine in Decomposing Tissues on the Development Rate of *Parasarcophaga ruficornis* (Diptera: Sarcophagidae) And Implications of This Effect on the Estimations of Post Mortem Intervals. *Journal of Forensic Sciences*, 37 (3): 867-872.

389. Chen WY, Hung TH, Shiao SF. (2004). Molecular identification of forensically important blow fly species (Diptera: Calliphoridae) in Taiwan. *J Med Entomol.*;41:47-57

390. Chophi R, Sharma S., Sharma S and Singh R (2019). Forensic entomotoxicology: current concepts, trends and challenges. *Journal of forensic and legal medicine*. 67, 28-36

391. Singh, R, Sharma P and Mehta R K (2012). Wildlife forensic entomology: A study on national level highlighted cases of tigers death in Ranthambour and Sariska national parks (Rajasthan) *J. Appl. Biosci.*,38(2): 127-131

392. Sperling, F. A., G. S. Anderson and D. A. Hickey (1994). A DNA-based approach to the identification of insect species used for postmorten interval estimation. *Journal of Forensic Science*39(2): 418-427.

393. Thyssen, P. J., A. C. Lessinger, A. M. Azeredo-Espin and A. X. Linhares (2005). The value of PCR-RFLP molecular markers for the differentiation of

immature stages of two necrophagous flies (Diptera: Calliphoridae) of potential forensic importance. *Neotropical* Entomology, 34(5): 777-783.

394. Jangir S and Sharma J D (2019). Molecular identification of carrion insects and their role in justice delivery system a thesis submitted to central university, Sagar, under University Grants Commission (Sodhganga)
395. Campobasso, C. P., F. A. Sperling, F. Introna, G. Di Vella, J. Hayes and J. D. Wells (2001). Human and insect mitochondrial DNA analysis from maggots. *Journal of Forensic Science*, 46(3): 685-687.
396. Wells, J. D., T. Pape and F. A. Sperling (2001). DNA-based identification and molecular systematics of forensically important Sarcophagidae (Diptera). *Journal of Forensic Science*, 46(5): 1098-1102
397. Hall, M.; Whitaker, A.; Richards, C. Forensic Entomology. In *The Forensic Ecology Handbook: From Crime Scene to Court*, 1st ed.; Marques-Grant, N., Roberts, J., Eds.; John Wiley and Sons Ltd.: Chichester, UK, 2012; pp. 111–140. ISBN 978-1-119-97419-2.
398. Amendt, J.; Campobasso, C.P.; Gaudry, E.; Reiter, C.; LeBlanc, H.N.; Hall, M. Best practice in forensic entomology—Standards and guidelines. *Int. J. Legal Med.* **2007**, *121*, 90–104.
399. James, S.H.; Nordby, J.J. *Forensic Science: An Introduction to Scientific and Investigative Techniques*, 3rd ed.; CRC Press: Boca Raton, FL, USA, 2002; ISBN 0-8493-1246-9.
400. Saks, M.J.; Koehler, J.J. The coming paradigm shift in forensic identification science. *Science* **2005**, *309*, 892–895.
401. Saferstein, R. *Criminalistics: An Introduction to Forensic Science*, 7th ed.; Prentice Hall: Upper Saddle River, NJ, USA, 2001.

402. Brettell, T.A.; Butler, J.M.; Saferstein, R. Forensic science. *Anal. Chem.* **2005**, *77*, 3839–3860.
403. Horswell, J. Crime Scene Investigation. In *The Practice of Crime Scene Investigation*, 1st ed.; CRC Press: Boca Raton, FL, USA, 2004.
404. Katz, E.; Halámek, J. Forensic science: A multidisciplinary approach. *J. Forensic Leg. Investig. Sci.* **2016**, *1*, 1–4.
405. Byrd, J.H.; Tomberlin, J.K. *Forensic Entomology: The Utility of Arthropods in Legal Investigations*, 3rd ed.; CRC Press: Boca Raton, FL, USA, 2020; ISBN 978-0-8153-5020-0.
406. Dadour, I.R.; Morris, B. Forensic Entomology: A Synopsis, Guide, and Update. In *Essentials of Autopsy Practice*, 1st ed.; Rutty, G.N., Ed.; Springer: London, UK, 2014; pp. 105–130.
407. Robinson, W.H. *Urban Insects and Arachnids: A Handbook of Urban Entomology*, 1st ed.; Cambridge University Press: Cambridge, UK, 2005; ISBN 9780521812535.
408. Bugelli, V.; Tarozzic, I.; Galante, N.; Bortolini, S.; Franceschetti, L. Review on forensic importance of myiasis: Focus on medicolegal issues on post-mortem interval estimation and neglect evaluation. *Legal Med.* **2023**, *63*, 102263.
409. Hagstrum, D.W.; Athanassiou, C.G. Improving stored product insect pest management: From theory to practice. *Insects* **2019**, *10*, 332.
410. Haines, A.M.; Webb, S.L.; Wallace, J.R. Conservation Forensics: The Intersection of Wildlife Crime, Forensics, and Conservation. In *Wildlife Biodiversity Conservation*, 1st ed.; Underkoffler, S.C., Adams, H.R., Eds.; Springer: Cham, Switzerland, 2021; pp. 125–146.

411. Matuszewski, S. Post-mortem interval estimation based on insect evidence: Current challenges. *Insects* **2021**, *12*, 314.
412. Bambaradeniya, Y.T.B.; Karunaratne, W.A.I.P.; Rakinawasam, S.V.; Tomberlin, J.K.; Goonerathne, I.; Kotakadeniya, R.B. Myiasis incidences reported in and around central province of Sri Lanka. *Int. J. Dermatol.* **2019**, *58*, 336–342.
413. Catts, E.P.; Goff, M.L. Forensic entomology in criminal investigations. *Annu. Rev. Entomol.* **1992**, *37*, 253–272.
414. Forbes, S.L.; Carter, D.O. Processes and Mechanisms of Death and Decomposition of Vertebrate Carrion. In *Carrion Ecology, Evolution, and Their Applications*, 1st ed.; Benbow, M.E., Tomberlin, J.K., Torone, A.M., Eds.; CRC Press: Boca Raton, FL, USA, 2015; pp. 13–30.
415. Payne, J.A.; King, E.W.; Beinhart, G. Arthropod succession and decomposition of buried pigs. *Nature* **1968**, *219*, 1180–1181.
416. Noriki, S.; Iino, S.; Kinoshita, K.; Fukazawa, Y.; Inai, K.; Sakai, T.; Kimura, H. Pathological analysis of cadavers for educational dissection by using postmortem imaging. *Pathol. Int.* **2019**, *69*, 580–600.
417. Bajerlein, D.; Taberski, D.; Matuszewski, S. Estimation of postmortem interval (PMI) based on empty puparia of *Phormia regina* (Meigen) (Diptera: Calliphoridae) and third larval stage of *Necrodes littoralis* (L.) (Coleoptera: Silphidae)–Advantages of using different PMI indicators. *J. Forensic Leg. Med.* **2018**, *55*, 95–98.
418. Pittner, S.; Bugelli, V.; Weitgasser, K.; Zissler, A.; Sanit, S.; Lutz, L.; Amendt, J. A field study to evaluate PMI estimation methods for advanced decomposition stages. *Int. J. Legal Med.* **2020**, *134*, 1361–1373.

419. Bambaradeniya, Y.T.B.; Magni, P.A.; Dadour, I.R. Current Status of Five Warm Season Diptera Species in Estimating the Post-Mortem Interval. *Ann. Entomol. Soc. Am.* **2023**, *116*, 19–50.
420. Kreitlow, K.L.T. Insect Succession in a Natural Environment. In *Forensic Entomology*, 2nd ed.; Byrd, J.H., Castner, J.L., Eds.; CRC Press: Boca Raton, FL, USA, 2009; pp. 251–269.
421. Amendt, J.; Richards, C.S.; Campobasso, C.P.; Zehner, R.; Hall, M.J. Forensic entomology: Applications and limitations. *Forensic Sci. Med. Pathol.* **2011**, *7*, 379–392.
422. Campobasso, C.P.; Di Vella, G.; Introna, F. Factors affecting decomposition and Diptera colonization. *Forensic Sci. Int.* **2001**, *120*, 18–27.
423. Kulshrestha, P.; Satpathy, D.K. Use of beetles in forensic entomology. *Forensic Sci. Int.* **2001**, *120*, 15–17.
424. Frost, C.L.; Braig, H.R.; Amendt, J.; Perotti, M.A. Indoor Arthropods of Forensic Importance: Insects Associated with Indoor Decomposition and Mites as Indoor Markers. In *Current Concepts in Forensic Entomology*, 1st ed.; Amendt, J., Goff, M.L., Campobasso, C.P., Grassberger, M., Eds.; Springer: Dordrecht, The Netherlands, 2010; pp. 93–108.
425. Vanin, S. Advances in Forensic Entomology in Missing Persons Investigations. In *Handbook of Missing Persons*, 1st ed.; Morewitz, S.J., Colls, C.S., Eds.; Springer: Cham, Switzerland, 2016; pp. 309–317.
426. Prasad, S.; Aneesh, E.M. Tools and techniques in forensic entomology—A critical review. *Int. J. Trop. Insect Sci.* **2020**, *42*, 2785–2794.
427. Charabidze, D.; Gosselin, M.; Hedouin, V. Use of necrophagous insects as evidence of cadaver relocation: Myth or reality? *Peer J.* **2017**, *5*, e3506.

428. Weatherbee, C.R.; Pechal, J.L.; Eric Benbow, M. The dynamic maggot mass microbiome. *Ann. Entomol. Soc. Am.* **2017**, *110*, 45–53.
429. Di Luise, E.; Magni, P.; Staiti, N.; Spitaleri, S.; Romano, C. Genotyping of human nuclear DNA recovered from the gut of fly larvae. *Forensic Sci. Int.* **2008**, *1*, 591–592.
430. Wells, J.D.; Stevens, J.R. Application of DNA-based methods in forensic entomology. *Annu. Rev. Entomol.* **2008**, *53*, 103–120.
431. Garrido-Cardenas, J.A.; Manzano-Agugliaro, F. The metagenomics worldwide research. *Curr. Genet.* **2017**, *63*, 819–829.
432. Roumpeka, D.D.; Wallace, R.J.; Escalettes, F.; Fotheringham, I.; Watson, M. A review of bioinformatics tools for bioprospecting from metagenomic sequence data. *Front. Genet.* **2017**, *8*, 23.
433. Carvalho, F.; Dadour, I.R.; Groth, D.M.; Harvey, M.L. Isolation and detection of ingested DNA from the immature stages of *Calliphora dubia* (Diptera: Calliphoridae) A forensically important blowfly. *Forensic Sci. Med. Pathol.* **2005**, *1*, 261–265.
434. Baqué, M.; Amendt, J.; Verhoff, M.A.; Zehner, R. Descriptive analyses of differentially expressed genes during larval development of *Calliphora vicina* (Diptera: Calliphoridae). *Int. J. Legal Med.* **2015**, *129*, 891–902.
435. Kintz, P.; Tracqui, A.; Ludes, B.; Waller, J.; Boukhabza, A.; Mangin, P.; Chaumont, A.J. Fly larvae and their relevance in forensic toxicology. *Am. J. Forensic Med. Pathol.* **1990**, *11*, 63–65.
436. Gosselin, M.; Wille, S.M.; Fernandez, M.D.M.R.; Di Fazio, V.; Samyn, N.; De Boeck, G.; Bourel, B. Entomotoxicology, experimental set-up and interpretation for forensic toxicologists. *Forensic Sci. Int.* **2011**, *208*, 1–9.

437. Stewart, M.A. The teaching of entomology. *J. Econ. Entomol.* **1929**, *22*, 777–781.
438. Morris, B.; Harvey, M.L.; Dadour, I.R. International Collaborations and Training. In *International Dimensions & Frontiers in Forensic Entomology*, 1st ed.; Tomberlin, J., Benbow, E., Eds.; CRC Press: Boca Raton, FL, USA, 2015; Volume 30, pp. 399–416.
439. Schoenly, K.G.; Haskell, N.H.; Mills, D.K.; Bieme-Ndi, C.; Larsen, K.; Lee, Y. Recreating death's acre in the school yard: Using pig carcasses as model corpses to teach concepts of forensic entomology & ecological succession. *Am. Biol. Teach.* **2006**, *68*, 402–410
440. Magni, P.; Guercini, S.; Leighton, A.; Dadour, I. Forensic entomologists: An evaluation of their status. *J. Insect Sci.* **2013**, *13*, 78.
441. Schoenly, K.G.; Michaud, J.P.; Moreau, G. Design and Analysis of Field Studies in Carrion Ecology. In *Carrion Ecology, Evolution, and Their Applications*, 1st ed.; Benbow, M.E., Tomberlin, J.K., Torone, A.M., Eds.; CRC Press: Boca Raton, FL, USA, 2015; pp. 129–148. ISBN 978-1-4665-7547-9.
442. Benbow, M.E.; Pechal, J.L. Forensic Entomology and the Microbiome. In *Forensic Entomology: The Utility of Arthropods in Legal Investigations*, 3rd ed.; Byrd, J.H., Tomberlin, J.K., Eds.; CRC Press: Boca Raton, FL, USA, 2020; pp. 499–517.
443. Michaud, J.P.; Schoenly, K.G.; Moreau, G. Rewriting ecological succession history: Did carrion ecologists get there first? *Q. Rev. Biol.* **2015**, *90*, 45–66.
444. Benecke, M.; Barksdale, L. Distinction of bloodstain patterns from fly artifacts. *Forensic Sci. Int.* **2003**, *137*, 152–159.

445. Dadour, I.R.; Cook, D.F.; Fissioli, J.N.; Bailey, W.J. Forensic entomology: Application, education and research in Western Australia. *Forensic Sci. Int.* **2001**, *120*, 48–52.
446. Archer, M.S.; Wallman, J.F. The development of forensic entomology in Australia and New Zealand: An overview of casework practice, quality control and standards. *Aust. J. Forensic Sci.* **2017**, *49*, 125–133.
447. Lutz, L.; Zehner, R.; Verhoff, M.A.; Bratzke, H.; Amendt, J. It is all about the insects: A retrospective on 20 years of forensic entomology highlights the importance of insects in legal investigations. *Int. J. Legal Med.* **2021**, *135*, 2637–2651.
448. Mégnin, P. *La faune des Cadavres. Application de l'entomologie a la Médicine Légal (Fauna of Cadavers. Application of Enomology in Legal Medicine)*; Encyclopdie scientifique des Aides-Mémoire; Les Belles Lettres: Paris, France, 1894; p. 214.
449. Payne, J.A. A summer carrion study of the baby pig Sus scrofa Linnaeus. *Ecology* **1965**, *46*, 592–602.
450. Tomberlin, J.K.; Mohr, R.; Benbow, M.E.; Tarone, A.M.; Vanlaerhoven, S. A roadmap for bridging basic and applied research in forensic entomology. *Annu. Rev. Entomol.* **2011**, *56*, 401–421.
451. Keh, B. Scope and applications of forensic entomology. *Annu. Rev. Entomol.* **1985**, *30*, 137–154.
452. Tomberlin, J.K.; Byrd, J.H.; Wallace, J.R.; Benbow, M.E. Assessment of decomposition studies indicates need for standardized and repeatable research methods in forensic entomology. *J. Forensic Res.* **2012**, *3*, 1000147.
453. Moreau, G. The pitfalls in the path of probabilistic inference in forensic entomology: A review. *Insects* **2021**, *12*, 240.

454. Gaudry, E.; Dourel, L. Forensic entomology: Implementing quality assurance for expertise work. *Int. J. legal Med.* **2013**, *127*, 1031–1037.
455. Magni, P.A.; Dadour, I. SmartInsects–Smartphone & Forensic Entomology. 2013 (Version 1.0). Mobile Application Software: IOS. Retrieved from App Store. Available online: https://apps.apple.com/us/app/smartinsects/id985074731 (accessed on 15 December 2022).
456. Campobasso, C.P.; Introna, F. The forensic entomologist in the context of the forensic pathologist's role. *Forensic Sci. Int.* **2001**, *120*, 132–139.
457. Amendt, J.; Krettek, R.; Niess, C.; Zehner, R.; Bratzke, H. Forensic entomology in Germany. *Forensic Sci. Int.* **2000**, *113*, 309–314.
458. Dolinski, C.; Shapiro-Ilan, D.; Lewis, E.E. Insect Cadaver Applications: Pros and Cons. In *Nematode Pathogenesis of Insects and Other Pests*, 1st ed.; Campos-Herrera, R., Ed.; Springer: Cham, Switzerland, 2015; pp. 207–229.
459. LeBlanc, H.N.; Logan, J.G. Exploiting Insect Olfaction in Forensic Entomology. In *Current Concepts in Forensic Entomology*, 1st ed.; Amendt, J., Goff, M.L., Campobasso, C.P., Grassberger, M., Eds.; Springer: Dordrecht, The Netherlands, 2009; pp. 205–221
460. Charabidze, D.; Depeme, A.; Devigne, C.; Hedouin, V. Do necrophagous blowflies (Diptera: Calliphoridae) lay their eggs in wounds?: Experimental data and implications for forensic entomology. *Forensic Sci. Int.* **2015**, *253*, 71–75.
461. Kinnaird, E.L. Decomposition and Insect Succession on Hanging Carcasses in Western Australia. Master by Research, The University of Western Australia, Perth, 3 November 2016. Available online: https://research-

repository.uwa.edu.au/en/publications/decomposition-and-insect-succession-on-hanging-carcasses-in-weste (accessed on 15 December 2022).

462. Bhadra, P.; Hart, A.J.; Hall, M.J.R. Factors affecting accessibility to blowflies of bodies disposed in suitcases. *Forensic Sci. Int.* **2014**, *239*, 62–72.
463. Wescott, D.J. Recent advances in forensic anthropology: Decomposition research. *Forensic Sci. Res.* **2018**, *3*, 278–293.
464. Finley, S.J.; Benbow, M.E.; Javan, G.T. Microbial communities associated with human decomposition and their potential use as postmortem clocks. *Int. J. Legal Med.* **2015**, *129*, 623–632.
465. Wallace, J.R. Aquatic Vertebrate Carrion Decomposition. In *Carrion Ecology, Evolution, and Their Applications*, 1st ed.; Benbow, M.E., Tomberlin, J.K., Torone, A.M., Eds.; CRC Press: Boca Raton, FL, USA, 2015; pp. 247–271.
466. Neven, L.G. Physiological responses of insects to heat. *Postharvest Biol. Technol.* **2000**, *21*, 103–111.
467. Sharanowski, B.J.; Walker, E.G.; Anderson, G.S. Insect succession and decomposition patterns on shaded and sunlit carrion in Saskatchewan in three different seasons. *Forensic Sci. Int.* **2008**, *179*, 219–240.
468. Bambaradeniya, Y.T.B.; Karunarathne, W.A.I.P.; Goonerathne, I.; Kotakadeniya, R.B.; Tomberlin, J.K. Use of development data to estimate colonization time of the myiasis-causing fly, *Chrysomya bezziana* (Diptera: Calliphoridae) collected from human wounds. *Sri Lanka J. Forensic Med. Sci. Law* **2016**, *7*, 19–26.
469. Iancu, L.; Dean, D.E.; Purcarea, C. Temperature influence on prevailing necrophagous Diptera and bacterial taxa with forensic implications for

postmortem interval estimation: A review. *J. Med. Entomol.* **2018**, *55*, 1369–1379.
470. Guo, J.; Fu, X.; Liao, H.; Hu, Z.; Long, L.; Yan, W.; Cai, J. Potential use of bacterial community succession for estimating post-mortem interval as revealed by high-throughput sequencing. *Sci. Rep.* **2016**, *6*, 24197.
471. Hofer, I.M.; Hart, A.J.; Martín-Vega, D.; Hall, M.J. Estimating crime scene temperatures from nearby meteorological station data. *Forensic Sci. Int.* **2020**, *306*, 110028.
472. Charabidze, D.; Hedouin, V. Temperature: The weak point of forensic entomology. *Int. J. Legal Med.* **2019**, *133*, 633–639.
473. Johnson, A.P.; Wallman, J.F.; Archer, M.S. Experimental and casework validation of ambient temperature corrections in forensic entomology. *J. Forensic Sci.* **2012**, *57*, 215–221.
474. Hofer, I.M.; Hart, A.J.; Martín-Vega, D.; Hall, M.J. Optimising crime scene temperature collection for forensic entomology casework. *Forensic Sci. Int.* **2017**, *270*, 129–138.
475. Turchetto, M.; Vanin, S. Climate Change and Forensic Entomology. In *Current Concepts in Forensic Entomology*, 1st ed.; Amendt, J., Goff, M.L., Campobasso, C.P., Grassberger, M., Eds.; Springer: Dordrecht, The Netherlands, 2009; pp. 327–351.
476. Michaud, J.P.; Schoenly, K.G.; Moreau, G. Sampling flies or sampling flaws? Experimental design and inference strength in forensic entomology. *J. Med. Entomol.* **2012**, *49*, 1–10.
477. Anderson, G.S.; Cervenka, V.J.; Haglund, W.; Sorg, M. Insects Associated with the Body: Their Use and Analyses. In *Advances in Forensic Taphonomy: Method, Theory, and Archaeological Perspectives*, 1st ed.;

Haglund, W.D., Sorg, M., Eds.; CRC Press: Boca Raton, FL, USA, 2002; p. 173200. ISBN 13: 978-14200-5835-2.

478. Touroo, R.; Fitch, A. Crime Scene Findings and the Identification, Collection, and Preservation of Evidence. In *Veterinary Forensic Pathology*, 1st ed.; Brooks, J.S., Ed.; Springer: Cham, Switzerland, 2018; pp. 9–25.

479. Mohr, R.M.; Tomberlin, J.K. Development and validation of a new technique for estimating a minimum postmortem interval using adult blow fly (Diptera: Calliphoridae) carcass attendance. *Int. J. Legal Med.* **2015**, *129*, 851–859.

480. Martín-Vega, D.; Hall, M.J.R. Estimating the age of *Calliphora vicina* eggs (Diptera: Calliphoridae): Determination of embryonic morphological landmarks and preservation of egg samples. *Int. J. Legal Med.* **2016**, *130*, 845–854.

481. Tyndale-Biscoe, M. Age-grading methods in adult insects: A review. *Bull. Entomol. Res.* **1984**, *74*, 341–377.

482. Firoozfar, F.; Moosa-Kazemi, H.; Baniardalani, M.; Abolhassani, M.; Khoobdel, M.; Rafinejd, J. Mass rearing of *Lucilia sericata Meigen* (Diptera: Calliphoridae). *Asian Pac. J. Trop. Biomed.* **2011**, *1*, 54–56.

483. Bilaniuk, V.; Beresford, D.V. Sampling adult blow flies (Diptera: Calliphoridae) at pig carcasses with sticky traps: Effects of trap colour, height, and inclination. *J. Can. Soc. Forensic Sci.* **2010**, *43*, 181–190.

484. Adams, Z.J.; Hall, M.J. Methods used for the killing and preservation of blowfly larvae, and their effect on post-mortem larval length. *Forensic Sci. Int.* **2003**, *138*, 50–61.

485. Davies, K.; Harvey, M.L. Internal morphological analysis for age estimation of blow fly pupae (Diptera: Calliphoridae) in postmortem interval estimation. *J. Forensic Sci.* **2013**, *58*, 79–84.
486. Brown, K.; Thorne, A.; Harvey, M. *Calliphora vicina* (Diptera: Calliphoridae) pupae: A timeline of external morphological development and a new age and PMI estimation tool. *Int. J. Legal Med.* **2015**, *129*, 835–850.
487. Weithmann, S.; von Hoermann, C.; Degasperi, G.; Brandt, K.; Steiger, S.; Ayasse, M. Temporal variability of the rove beetle (Coleoptera: Staphylinidae) community on small vertebrate carrion and its potential use for forensic entomology. *Forensic Sci. Int.* **2021**, *323*, 110792.]
488. Dalal, J.; Sharma, S.; Bhardwaj, T.; Dhattarwal, S.K. Assessment of post-mortem submersion interval using total aquatic decomposition scores of drowned human cadavers. *J. Forensic. Sci.* **2023**, *68*, 549–557.
489. Rivers, D.B.; Dahlem, G.A. *The Science of Forensic Entomology*, 2nd ed.; John Wiley & Sons: Toronto, ON, Canada, 2023; ISBN 97811199403664.
490. Stamper, T.; Weidner, L.; Nigoghosian, G.; Johnson, N.; Wang, C.; Levesque-Bristol, C. Towards understanding how to instruct students in dichotomous identification keys in a mixed STEM forensic science education environment. *JFSE* **2020**, *2*, 1.
491. Drijfhout, F.P. Cuticular Hydrocarbons: A New Tool in Forensic Entomology? In *Current Concepts in Forensic Entomology*, 1st ed.; Amendt, J., Goff, M.L., Campobasso, C.P., Grassberger, M., Eds.; Springer: Dordrecht, The Netherlands, 2009.
492. Pechal, J.L.; Moore, H.; Drijfhout, F.; Benbow, M.E. Hydrocarbon profiles throughout adult Calliphoridae aging: A promising tool for forensic entomology. *Forensic Sci. Int.* **2014**, *245*, 65–71.

493. Sukontason, K.; Sukontason, K.L.; Boonchu, N.; Chaiwong, T.; Piangjai, S. Ultrastructure of eggshell of *Chrysomya nigripes Aubertin* (Diptera: Calliphoridae). *Parasitol. Res.* **2004**, *93*, 151–154.

494. Velásquez, Y.; Magaña, C.; Martínez-Sánchez, A.; Rojo, S. Diptera of forensic importance in the Iberian Peninsula: Larval identification key. *Med. Vet. Entomol.* **2010**, *24*, 293–308.

495. James, M.T. *The Flies That Cause Myiasis in Man*; US Department of Agriculture, Government Printing Office: Washington, DC, USA, 1947.

496. Zumpt, F. *Myiasis in Man and Animals in the Old World: A Textbook for Physicians, Veterinarians and Zoologists*; Butterworth & Co., Ltd.: London, UK, 1965.

497. Smith, K.V.G. *A Manual of Forensic Entomology*, 1st ed.; Department of Entomology, British Museum: London, UK, 1986; ISBN 9780565009908.

498. Wood, D.M.; Borkent, A. Phylogeny and Classification of the Nematocera. In *Manual of Nearctic Diptera*, 1st ed.; McAlpine, J.F., Wood, D.M., Eds.; Research Branch Agriculture Canada Monograph No. 32; Canadian Government Publishing Centre: Hull, QC, Canada, 1989; pp. 1333–1370.

499. Carvalho, C.J.B.D.; Mello-Patiu, C.A.D. Chave de identificação para as espécies comuns de Diptera da América do Sul de interesse forense. *Rev. Bras. Entomol.* **2008**, *52*, 390–406.

500. Szpila, K.; Richet, R.; Pape, T. Third instar larvae of flesh flies (Diptera: Sarcophagidae) of forensic importance—Critical review of characters and key for European species. *Parasitol. Res.* **2015**, *114*, 2279–2289.

501. Whitworth, T. Keys to the Genera and Species of Blow Flies (Diptera: Calliphoridae) of America, North of Mexico. In *Forensic Entomology: The*

Utility of Arthropods in Legal Investigations, 3rd ed.; Byrd, J.H., Tomberlin, J.K., Eds.; CRC Press: Boca Raton, FL, USA, 2020; pp. 413–443.

502. Wallman, J.F. A key to the adults of species of blowflies in southern Australia known or suspected to breed in carrion. *Med. Vet. Entomol.* **2001**, *15*, 433–437.

503. Hanley, G.A.; Cuthrell, D.L. *The Carrion Beetles of North Dakota, Including Species Descriptions and Identification Keys for the Entire North American Silphid Fauna*; Minot State University: Minot, ND, USA, 2010.

504. Brunke, A.; Newton, A.; Klimaszewski, J.; Majka, C.; Marshall, S. Staphylinidae of eastern Canada and adjacent United States. Key to subfamilies: Staphylininae: Tribes and subtribes, and species of Staphylinina. *Can. J. Arthropod Identif.* **2011**, *12*, 1–110.

505. Mendonça, P.M.; dos Santos-Mallet, J.R.; de Mello, R.P.; Gomes, L.; de Carvalho Queiroz, M.M. Identification of fly eggs using scanning electron microscopy for forensic investigations. *Micron* **2008**, *39*, 802–807.

506. Ubero-Pascal, N.; Arnaldos, I.; López-Esclapez, R.; García, M.D. Microscopy and forensic entomology. *Microsc. Sci. Technol. Appl. Educ. Microsc. Book Ser.* **2010**, *4*, 1548–1556.

507. Grzywacz, A. Third instar larva morphology of *Hydrotaea cyrtoneurina* (Zetterstedt, 1845) (Diptera: Muscidae)-a species of forensic interest. *Pol. J. Entomol.* **2013**, *82*, 303–315.

508. Hore, G.; Maity, A.; Naskar, A.; Ansar, W.; Ghosh, S.; Saha, G.K.; Banerjee, D. Scanning electron microscopic studies on antenna of *Hemipyrellia ligurriens* (Wiedemann, 1830) (Diptera: Calliphoridae)—A blow fly species of forensic importance. *Acta Trop.* **2017**, *172*, 20–28.

509. Giglio, A.; Ferrero, E.A.; Perrotta, E.; Tripepi, S.; Brandmayr, T.Z. Ultrastructure and comparative morphology of mouth-part sensilla in ground beetle larvae (Insecta, Coleoptera, Carabidae). *Zool. Anz.* **2003**, *242*, 277–292.

510. Ortloff, A.; Zanetti, N.; Centeno, N.; Silva, R.; Bustamante, F.; Olave, A. Ultramorphological characteristics of mature larvae of *Nitidula carnaria* (Schaller 1783) (Coleoptera: Nitidulidae), a beetle species of forensic importance. *Forensic Sci. Int.* **2014**, *239*, e1–e9.

511. Chen, W.Y.; Hung, T.H.; Shiao, S.F. Molecular identification of forensically important blow fly species (Diptera: Calliphoridae) in Taiwan. *J. Med. Entomol.* **2004**, *41*, 47–57.

512. Batovska, J.; Blacket, M.J.; Brown, K.; Lynch, S.E. Molecular identification of mosquitoes (Diptera: Culicidae) in southeastern Australia. *Ecol. Evol.* **2016**, *6*, 3001–3011.

513. Magni, P.A.; Harvey, M.L.; Saravo, L.; Dadour, I.R. Entomological evidence: Lessons to be learnt from a cold case review. *Forensic Sci. Int.* **2012**, *223*, 31–34.

514. Rolo, E.S.A. DNA Barcoding and Forensic Entomology: A Molecular Approach for Diptera Species' Identification. Ph.D. Thesis, University of Lisbon, Lisboa, Portugal, 2010. Available online: **https://hdl.handle.net/10451/2024** (accessed on 15 December 2022).

515. Boehme, P.; Amendt, J.; Disney, R.H.L.; Zehner, R. Molecular identification of carrion-breeding scuttle flies (Diptera: Phoridae) using COI barcodes. *Int. J. Legal Med.* **2010**, *124*, 577–581.

516. Stevens, J.; Wall, R. Genetic relationships between blowflies (Calliphoridae) of forensic importance. *Forensic Sci. Int.* **2001**, *120*, 116–123.
517. Wallman, J.F.; Leys, R.; Hogendoorn, K. Molecular systematics of Australian carrion-breeding blowflies (Diptera: Calliphoridae) based on mitochondrial DNA. *Invertebr. Syst.* **2005**, *19*, 1–15.
518. Harvey, M.L.; Dadour, I.R.; Gaudieri, S. Mitochondrial DNA cytochrome oxidase I gene: Potential for distinction between immature stages of some forensically important fly species (Diptera) in western Australia. *Forensic Sci. Int.* **2003**, *131*, 134–139.
519. Harvey, M.L.; Mansell, M.W.; Villet, M.H.; Dadour, I.R. Molecular identification of some forensically important blowflies of southern Africa and Australia. *Med. Vet. Entomol.* **2003**, *17*, 363–369.
520. Harvey, M.L.; Gaudieri, S.; Villet, M.H.; Dadour, I.R. A global study of forensically significant calliphorids: Implications for identification. *Forensic Sci. Int.* **2008**, *177*, 66–76.
521. Day, D.M.; Wallman, J.F. Width as an alternative measurement to length for post-mortem interval estimations using *Calliphora augur* (Diptera: Calliphoridae) larvae. *Forensic Sci. Int.* **2006**, *159*, 158–167.
522. Hu, Y.; Yuan, X.; Zhu, F.; Lei, C. Development time and size-related traits in the oriental blowfly, *Chrysomya megacephala* along a latitudinal gradient from China. *J. Therm. Bio.* **2010**, *35*, 366–371.
523. Zhang, Y.; Wang, Y.; Yang, L.; Tao, L.; Wang, J. Development of *Chrysomya megacephala* at constant temperatures within its colony range in Yangtze River Delta region of China. *Forensic Sci. Res.* **2018**, *3*, 74–82.
524. Bambaradeniya, Y.T.B.; Karunaratne, W.I.P.; Tomberlin, J.K.; Goonerathne, I.; Kotakadeniya, R.B.; Magni, P.A. Effect of temperature and tissue type on

the development of the forensic fly *Chrysomya megacephala* (Diptera: Calliphoridae). *J. Med. Entomol.* **2019**, *56*, 1571–1581.

525. Hu, G.; Wang, Y.; Sun, Y.; Zhang, Y.; Wang, M.; Wang, J. Development of *Chrysomya rufifacies* (Diptera: Calliphoridae) at constant temperatures within its colony range in Yangtze River Delta Region of China. *J. Med. Entomol.* **2019**, *56*, 1215–1224.
526. Bambaradeniya, Y.T.B.; Karunaratne, W.A.I.P.; Tomberlin, J.K.; Magni, P.A. Effect of type of tissue on the development of *Chrysomya rufifacies* (Diptera: Calliphoridae) in Sri Lanka. *J. Med. Entomol.* **2021**, *58*, 1673–1679.
527. Bambaradeniya, Y.T.B.; Karunaratne, W.A.I.P.; Tomberlin, J.K.; Goonerathne, I.; Kotakadeniya, R.B. Effect of temperature and tissue type on the development of myiasis causing fly; *Chrysomya bezziana* (Diptera: Calliphoridae). *J. Med. Entomol.* **2019**, *56*, 625–631.
528. Grassberger, M.; Reiter, C. Effect of temperature on *Lucilia sericata* (Diptera: Calliphoridae) development with special reference to the isomegalen-and isomorphen-diagram. *Forensic Sci. Int.* **2001**, *120*, 32–36.
529. Bambaradeniya, Y.T.B.; Karunaratne, W.I.P.; Tomberlin, J.K.; Goonerathne, I.; Kotakadeniya, R.B. Temperature and tissue type impact development of *Lucilia cuprina* (Diptera: Calliphoridae) in Sri Lanka. *J. Med. Entomol.* **2018**, *55*, 285–291.
530. Ma, T.; Huang, J.; Wang, J.F. Study on the pupal morphogenesis of *Chrysomya rufifacies* (Macquart) (Diptera: Calliphoridae) for postmortem interval estimation. *Forensic Sci. Int.* **2015**, *253*, 88–93.

531. Feng, D.X.; Liu, G.C. Pupal age estimation of forensically important *Megaselia spiracularis* Schmitz (Diptera: Phoridae). *Forensic Sci. Int.* **2013**, *231*, 199–203.
532. Feng, D.X.; Liu, G.C. Pupal age estimation of forensically important *Megaselia scalaris* (Loew) (Diptera: Phoridae). *Forensic Sci. Int.* **2014**, *236*, 133–137.
533. Li, L.; Wang, J.; Wang, Y. A comparative study of the decomposition of pig carcasses in a methyl methacrylate box and open-air conditions. *J. Forensic Legal Med.* **2016**, *42*, 92–95.
534. Nur Aliah, N.A.; Heo, C.C.; Noor Shafini, M.; Mohd Hafizi, M. Age estimation of forensically important blowfly, *Chrysomya megacephala* (Diptera: Calliphoridae) pupae using micro-computed tomography imaging. *Trop. Biomed.* **2019**, *36*, 640–653.
535. Feng, D.X.; Wu, J.; Sun, D.P. Intrapuparial age estimation of forensically important *Dohrniphora cornuta* (Diptera: Phoridae). *J. Med. Entomol.* **2021**, *58*, 616–624.
536. Voss, S.C.; Magni, P.; Dadour, I.; Nansen, C. Reflectance-based determination of age and species of blowfly puparia. *Int. J. Legal Med.* **2017**, *131*, 263–274.
537. Brown, K.; Harvey, M. Optical coherence tomography: Age estimation of *Calliphora vicina* pupae in vivo? *Forensic Sci. Int.* **2014**, *242*, 157–161.
538. Moore, H.E.; Adam, C.D.; Drijfhout, F.P. Potential Use of Hydrocarbons for Aging *Lucilia sericata* Blowfly Larvae to Establish the Postmortem Interval. *J. Forensic Sci.* **2013**, *58*, 404–412.
539. Frederickx, C.; Dekeirsschieter, J.; Brostaux, Y.; Wathelet, J.P.; Verheggen, F.J.; Haubruge, E. Volatile organic compounds released by blowfly larvae

and pupae: New perspectives in forensic entomology. *Forensic Sci. Int.* **2012**, *219*, 215–220.

540. Yanmanee, S.; Husemann, M.; Benbow, M.E.; Suwannapong, G. Larval development rates of *Chrysomya rufifacies Macquart*, 1842 (Diptera: Calliphoridae) within its native range in South-East Asia. *Forensic Sci. Int.* **2016**, *266*, 63–67.
541. Van der Merwe, S.S. The Identification of Diptera of the Grave and Their Succession Patterns during Winter and Summer in Central South Africa, with Reference to Forensic Applications. Ph.D. Thesis, University of the Free State, Bloemfontein, South Africa, 2016. Available online: **http://hdl.handle.net/11660/4033** (accessed on 2 May 2023).
542. Swiger, S.L.; Hogsette, J.A.; Butler, J.F. Laboratory colonization of the blow flies, *Chrysomya megacephala* (Diptera: Calliphoridae) and *Chrysomya rufifacies* (Diptera: Calliphoridae). *J. Econ. Entomol.* **2014**, *107*, 1780–1784.
543. Archer, M.S.; Jones, S.D.; Wallman, J.F. Delayed reception of live blowfly (*Calliphora vicina* and *Chrysomya rufifacies*) larval samples: Implications for minimum postmortem interval estimates. *Forensic Sci. Res.* **2018**, *3*, 27–39.
544. Pounder, D.J. Forensic entomo-toxicology. *J. Forensic Sci. Soc.* **1991**, *31*, 469–472.
545. Introna, F.; Campobasso, C.P.; Goff, M.L. Entomotoxicology. *Forensic Sci. Int.* **2001**, *120*, 42–47.
546. Scott, A.M. Crime Scene Documentation. In *Wiley Encyclopedia of Forensic Science*, 1st ed.; Jamieson, A., Moenssens, A., Eds.; John Wiley and Sons: Hoboken, NJ, USA, 2009.

547. Byrd, J.; Sutton, L. Forensic entomology for the investigator. *Wiley Interdiscip. Rev. Forensic Sci.* **2020**, *2*, 1370.
548. Miller, M.T. Crime Scene Investigation. In *Forensic Science: An Introduction to Scientific and Investigative Techniques*, 1st ed.; James, S.H., Nordby, J.J., Eds.; CRC Press: Boca Raton, FL, USA, 2002; pp. 143–164.
549. Hall, M.J.R. The relationship between research and casework in forensic entomology. *Insects* **2021**, *12*, 174.
550. Krinsky, W.L. Forensic Entomology. *Med. Vet. Entomol.* **2019**, *5*, 51–60. [
551. Weidner, L.M.; Meeds, A.W.; Noblesse, A.P.; Hans, K.R. A review of Forensic Entomology literature in the southwestern United States. *Wiley Interdiscip. Rev. Forensic Sci.* **2021**, *3*, e1421.
552. Niederegger, S.; Pastuschek, J.; Mall, G. Preliminary studies of the influence of fluctuating temperatures on the development of various forensically relevant flies. *Forensic Sci. Int.* **2010**, *199*, 72–78.
553. Wang, Y.; Li, L.L.; Wang, J.F.; Wang, M.; Yang, L.J.; Tao, L.Y.; Hou, Z.L. Development of the green bottle fly *Lucilia illustris* at constant temperatures. *Forensic Sci. Int.* **2016**, *267*, 136–144.
554. Greenberg, B.; Tantawi, T.I. Different developmental strategies in two boreal blow flies (Diptera: Calliphoridae). *J. Med. Entomol.* **1993**, *30*, 481–484.
555. Ames, C.; Turner, B. Low temperature episodes in development of blowflies: Implications for postmortem interval estimation. *Med. Vet. Entomol.* **2003**, *17*, 178–186.
556. Ireland, S.; Turner, B. The effects of larval crowding and food type on the size and development of the blowfly, *Calliphora vomitoria*. *Forensic Sci. Int.* **2006**, *159*, 175–181.

557. Niederegger, S.; Wartenberg, N.; Spiess, R.; Mall, G. Influence of food substrates on the development of the blowflies *Calliphora vicina* and *Calliphora vomitoria* (Diptera, Calliphoridae). *Parasitol. Res.* **2013**, *112*, 2847–2853.
558. Wood, T.; Pyper, K.; Casali, F. Effects of cocaine and heroin, and their combination, on the development rate of *Calliphora vomitoria* (Diptera: Calliphoridae). *Sci. Justice* **2022**, *62*, 471–475
559. Donovan, S.E.; Hall, M.J.R.; Turner, B.D.; Moncrieff, C.B. Larval growth rates of the blowfly, *Calliphora vicina*, over a range of temperatures. *Med. Vet. Entomol.* **2006**, *20*, 106–114.
560. Hwang, C.C.; Turner, B.D. Small-scaled geographical variation in life-history traits of the blowfly *Calliphora vicina* between rural and urban populations. *Entomol. Exp. Appl.* **2009**, *132*, 218–224.
561. Aak, A.; Birkemoe, T.; Leinaas, H.P. Phenology and life history of the blowfly *Calliphora vicina* in stockfish production areas. *Entomol. Exp. Appl.* **2011**, *139*, 35–46.
562. Sanei-Dehkordi, A.; Khamesipour, A.; Akbarzadeh, K.; Akhavan, A.A.; Rassi, Y.; Oshaghi, M.A.; Rafinejad, J. Experimental colonization and life table of the *Calliphora vicina* (Robineau-Desvoidy) (Diptera: Calliphoridae). *J. Entomol. Zool. Stud.* **2014**, *2*, 45–48.
563. Baqué, M.; Filmann, N.; Verhoff, M.A.; Amendt, J. Establishment of developmental charts for the larvae of the blow fly *Calliphora vicina* using quantile regression. *Forensic Sci. Int.* **2015**, *248*, 1–9.
564. Byrd, J.H.; Allen, J.C. The development of the black blow fly, *Phormia regina* (Meigen). *Forensic Sci. Int.* **2001**, *120*, 79–88.

565. Nabity, P.D.; Higley, L.G.; Heng-Moss, T.M. Light-induced variability in development of forensically important blow fly *Phormia regina* (Diptera: Calliphoridae). *J. Med. Entomol.* **2007**, *44*, 351–358.
566. Roe, A.L. Development Modeling of *Lucilia sericata* and *Phormia regina* (Diptera: Calliphoridae). Ph.D. Thesis, University of Nebraska-Lincoin, Lincoln, NE, USA, 2014.
567. Roe, A.L.; Higley, L.G. Stage Transitions in *Lucilia sericata* and *Phormia regina* (Diptera: Calliphoridae) and Implications for Forensic Science. *Insects* **2023**, *14*, 315.
568. Sukhapanth, N.; Upatham, E.S.; Ketavan, C. Effects of feed and media on egg production, growth and survivorship of flies (Diptera: Calliphoridae, Muscidae and Sarcophagidae). *J. Sci. Soc. Thailand* **1988**, *14*, 41–50.
569. Amoudi, M.A.; Diab, F.M.; Abou-Fannah, S.S. Development rate and mortality of immature *Parasarcophaga* (Liopygia) *ruficornis* (Diptera: Sarcophagidae) at constant laboratory temperatures. *J. Med. Entomol.* **1994**, *31*, 168–170.
570. Nassu, M.P.; Thyssen, P.J.; Linhares, A.X. Developmental rate of immatures of two fly species of forensic importance: *Sarcophaga* (Liopygia) *ruficornis* and *Microcerella halli* (Diptera: Sarcophagidae). *Parasitol. Res.* **2014**, *113*, 217–222.
571. Adhikari, K.; Khanikor, B.; Sarma, R.; Mahanta, S.; Kalita, J. Study on the life history and protein content of *Sarcophaga ruficornis* (Diptera: Sarcophagidiae) a forensically important insect. *J. Zool. Stud.* **2016**, *3*, 1–8.
572. Bansode, S.A.; More, V.R.; Zambare, S.P. Effect of Constant Temperature (20 °C, 25 °C, 30 °C, 35 °C, 40 °C) on the Development of Sarcophagidae:

Diptera (FAB) (Sarcophagidae: Diptera). *J. Pet. Environ. Biotechnol.* **2016**, *7*, 2.

573. Barbosa, T.M.; Cruz, M.R.P.; Pontes, W.J.T.; Vasconcelos, S.D. Aspects of the reproductive behaviour and development of two forensically relevant species, *Blaesoxipha (Gigantotheca) stallengi* (Lahille, 1907) and *Sarcophaga (Liopygia) ruficornis* (Fabricius, 1794) (Diptera: Sarcophagidae). *Rev. Bras. Entomol.* **2019**, *63*, 124–129.
574. Prawirodisastro, M.; Benjamin, D.M. Laboratory study on the biology and ecology of *Megaselia scalaris* (Diptera: Phoridae). *J. Med. Entomol.* **1979**, *16*, 317–320.
575. Trumble, J.T.; Pienkowski, R.L. Development and survival of *Megaselia scalaris* (Diptera: Phoridae) at selected temperatures and photoperiods. *Proc. Entomol. Soc. Wash.* **1979**, *81*, 207–210.
576. Greenberg, B.; Wells, J.D. Forensic use of *Megaselia abdita* and *M. scalaris* (Phoridae: Diptera): Case studies, development rates, and egg structure. *J. Med. Entomol.* **1998**, *35*, 205–209.
577. Harrison, D.A.; Cooper, R.L. Characterization of development, behavior and neuromuscular physiology in the phorid fly, *Megaselia scalaris*. *Comp. Biochem. Physiol. Part A Mol. Integr. Physiol.* **2003**, *136*, 427–439.
578. Zuha, R.M.; Razak, T.A.; Ahmad, N.W.; Omar, B. Interaction effects of temperature and food on the development of forensically important fly, *Megaselia scalaris* (Loew) (Diptera: Phoridae). *Parasitol. Res.* **2012**, *111*, 2179–2187.
579. Zuha, R.M.; Omar, B. Developmental rate, size, and sexual dimorphism of *Megaselia scalaris* (Loew) (Diptera: Phoridae): Its possible implications in forensic entomology. *Parasitol. Res.* **2014**, *113*, 2285–2294.

580. Chakraborty, A.; Naskar, A.; Parui, P.; Banerjee, D. Developmental variation of Indian thermophilic variety of scuttle fly *Megaselia* (Megaselia) *scalaris* (Loew, 1866) (Diptera: Phoridae) on different substrates. *Scientifica* **2016**, *2016*, 4257081
581. Thomas, J.K.; Sanford, M.R.; Longnecker, M.; Tomberlin, J.K. Effects of temperature and tissue type on the development of *Megaselia scalaris* (Diptera: Phoridae). *J. Med. Entomol.* **2016**, *53*, 519–525.
582. Ong, S.Q.; Ahmad, H.; Tan, E.H. Substrate moisture affects the development of *Megaselia scalaris* (Diptera: Phoridae): An implication of the growth circumstances of the fly in forensic entomology. *Environ. Entomol.* **2018**, *47*, 1582–1585.
583. Castillo-Alanis, L.A.; González-Hernández, A.E.; Quijano-Mateos, A.; Pedraza-Lara, C.S.; Villavicencio-Queijeiro, A.; Bravo-Gómez, M.E. Standardization of a Culture Medium for *Megaselia scalaris* (Diptera: Phoridae) for Entomotoxicological Studies. *J. Med. Entomol.* **2020**, *57*, 1421–1431.
584. Matuszewski, S.; Hall, M.J.; Moreau, G.; Schoenly, K.G.; Tarone, A.M.; Villet, M.H. Pigs vs people: The use of pigs as analogues for humans in forensic entomology and taphonomy research. *Int. J. Legal Med.* **2020**, *134*, 793–810.
585. Voss, S.C.; Cook, D.F.; Dadour, I.R. Decomposition and insect succession of clothed and unclothed carcasses in Western Australia. *Forensic Sci. Int.* **2011**, *211*, 67–75.
586. Kotzé, Z.; Aimar, S.; Amendt, J.; Anderson, G.S.; Bourguignon, L.; Hall, M.J.; Tomberlin, J.K. The forensic entomology case report—A global perspective. *Insects* **2021**, *12*, 283.

587. Tilstone, W.J.; Hastrup, M.L.; Hald, C. *Fisher's Techniques of Crime Scene Investigation, First International Edition*; CRC Press: Boca Raton, FL, USA, 2012.
588. Smith, K.G.V. *A Manual of Forensic Entomology*; Cornell University Press: Ithaca, NY, USA, 1986.
589. Amendt, J.; Richards, C.S.; Campobasso, C.P.; Zehner, R.; Hall, M.J.R. Forensic entomology: Applications and limitations. *Forensic Sci. Med. Pathol.* **2011**, *7*, 379–392.
590. de Carvahlo, L.M.L. Toxicology and forensic entomology. In *Current Concept in Forensic Entomology*; Amendt, J., Goff, M.L., Grassberger, M., Campobasso, C.P., Eds.; Springer: Berlin/Heidelberg, Germany, 2010; pp. 163–178.
591. Marchetti, D.; Arena, E.; Boschi, I.; Vanin, S. Human DNA extraction from empty puparia. *Forensic Sci. Int.* **2013**, *229*, e26–e29.
592. Mukherjee, S.; Singh, P.; Tuccia, F.; Pradelli, J.; Giordani, G.; Vanin, S. DNA characterization from gut content of larvae of *Megaselia scalaris* (Diptera, Phoridae). *Sci. Justice* **2019**, *59*, 654–659.
593. Miller, M.L.; Lord, W.D.; Goff, M.L.; Donnelly, B.; McDonough, E.T.; Alexis, J.C. Isolation of amitriptyline and nortriptyline from fly puparia (Phoridae) and beetle exuviae (Dermestidae) associated with mummified human remains. *J. Forensic Sci.* **1994**, *39*, 1305–1313.
594. Grassberger, M.; Reiter, C. Effect of temperature on *Lucilia sericata* (Diptera: Calliphoridae) development with special reference to the isomegalen- and isomorphen-diagram. *Forensic Sci. Int.* **2001**, *120*, 32–36.
595. Richards, C.S.; Paterson, I.D.; Villet, M.H. Estimating the age of immature *Chrysomya albiceps* (Diptera: Calliphoridae), correcting for

temperature and geographical latitude. *Int. J. Leg. Med.* **2008**, *122*, 271–279.

596. Charabidze, D.; Gosselin, M.; Hedouin, V. Use of necrophagous insects as evidence of cadaver relocation: Myth or reality? *PeerJ* **2017**, *5*, e3506.
597. Vanin, S.; Tasinato, P.; Ducolin, G.; Terranova, C.; Zancaner, S.; Montisci, M.; Ferrara, P.; Turchetto, M. Use of *Lucilia* species (Diptera: Calliphoridae) for forensic investigations in Southern Europe. *Forensic Sci Int.* **2008**, *177*, 37–41.
598. Lo Pinto, S.; Giordani, G.; Tuccia, F.; Ventura, F.; Vanin, S. First records of *Synthesiomyia nudiseta* (Diptera: Muscidae) from forensic cases in Italy. *Forensic Sci. Inter.* **2017**, *276*, e1–e7.
599. Turchetto, M.; Vanin, S. Forensic Entomology and Climatic Change. *Forensic Sci. Inter.* **2004**, *146*, 207–209.
600. The International Code of Zoological Nomenclature. Available online: **https://www.iczn.org/the-code/the-international-code-of-zoological-nomenclature/** (accessed on 1 July 2024).
601. Grzywacz, A.; Hall, M.J.; Pape, T.; Szpila, K. Muscidae (Diptera) of forensic importance-an identification key to third instar larvae of the Western Palaearctic region and a catalogue of the muscid carrion community. *Int. J. Legal Med.* **2017**, *131*, 855–866.
602. Rozkošný, R.; Gregor, F.; Pont, A.C. The European Fanniidae (Diptera). *Acta Sci. Nat. Brno* **1997**, *31*, 1–80.
603. Szpila, K. Key for the identification of third instars of European blowflies (Diptera: Calliphoridae) of forensic importance. In *Current Concepts in Forensic Entomology*; Amendt, J., Goff, M.L., Campobasso, P.C.,

Grassberger, M., Eds.; Springer: Dordrecht, The Netherlands, 2010; pp. 43–56.

604. Szpila, K.; Richet, R.; Pape, T. Third instar larvae of flesh flies (Diptera: Sarcophagidae) of forensic importance—Critical review of characters and key for European species. *Parasitol. Res.* **2015**, *114*, 2279–2289.

605. Erzinçlioğlu, Y.Z. Immature stages of British *Calliphora* and *Cynomya*, with a re-evaluation of the taxonomic characters of larval Calliphoridae (Diptera). *J. Nat. Hist.* **1985**, *19*, 69–96.

606. Skidmore, P. *The Biology of the Muscidae of the World*; Springer: Dordrecht, The Netherlands, 1985.

607. Giordani, G.; Grzywacz, A.; Vanin, S. Characterization and identification of puparia of *Hydrotaea* Robineau-Desvoidy, 1830 (Diptera: Muscidae) from forensic and archaeological contexts. *J. Med. Entomol.* **2018**, *56*, 45–54.

608. Giordani, G.; Tuccia, F.; Floris, I.; Vanin, S. First record of *Phormia regina* (Meigen, 1826) (Diptera: Calliphoridae) from mummies at the Sant'Antonio Abate Cathedral of Castelsardo, Sardinia, Italy. *PeerJ* **2018**, *6*, e4176.

609. Giordani, G.; Tuccia, F.; Zoppis, S.; Vecchiotti, C.; Vanin, S. Record of *Leptometopa latipes* (Diptera: Milichiidae) from a human cadaver in the Mediterranean area. *Forensic Sci. Res.* **2018**, *3*, 94–102.

610. Giordani, G.; Tuccia, F.; Martín-Vega, D.; Angell, C.S.; Pradelli, J.; Vanin, S. Morphological and molecular characterization of puparia of Piophilidae species of forensic relevance. *Med. Vet. Entomol.* **2023**, *37*, 339–358.

611. Giordani, G.; Vanin, S. Morphological characterization of puparia and molecular analysis of *Heleomyza serrata* (Linnaeus, 1758) (Diptera:

Heleomyzidae): A species of potential forensic interest. *Eur. J. Zool.* **2023**, *90*, 604–613.
612. Scaramozzino, P.L.; Di Giovanni, F.; Loni, A.; Gisondi, S.; Lucchi, A.; Cerretti, P. Tachinid (Diptera, Tachinidae) parasitoids of *Lobesia botrana* (Denis & Schiffermüller, 1775) (Lepidoptera, Tortricidae) and other moths. *ZooKeys* **2020**, *934*, 111–140.
613. Wells, J.; Stevens, J. Application of DNA-based methods in forensic entomology. *Annu. Rev. Entomol.* **2008**, *53*, 103–120.
614. Mazzanti, M.; Alessandrini, F.; Tagliabracci, A.; Wells, J.D.; Campobasso, C.P. DNA degradation and genetic analysis of empty puparia: Genetic identification limits in forensic entomology. *Forensic Sci. Int.* **2010**, *195*, 99–102.
615. Moore, H.E.; Pechal, J.L.; Benbow, M.E.; Drijfhout, F.P. The potential use of cuticular hydrocarbons and multivariate analysis to age empty puparial cases of *Calliphora vicina* and *Lucilia sericata*. *Sci. Rep.* **2017**, *7*, 1933.
616. Martín-Vega, D.; Hall, M.J.; Simonsen, T.J. Resolving confusion in the use of concepts and terminology in intrapuparial development studies of cyclorrhaphous Diptera. *J. Med. Entomol.* **2016**, *53*, 1249–1251.
617. Vanin, S.; Huchet, J. Forensic Entomology and Funerary Archaeoentomology. In *Taphonomy of Human Remains: Analysis of the Death and the Depositional Environments*; Schotsmans, E., Marquez-Grant, N., Forbes, S., Eds.; John Wiley & Sons Ltd.: Oxford, UK, 2017; pp. 176–186.
618. Martín-Vega, D.; Baz, A.; Díaz-Aranda, L.M. The immature stages of the necrophagous fly, *Prochyliza nigrimana*: Comparison with *Piophila*

casei and medicolegal considerations (Diptera: Piophilidae). *Parasitol. Res.* **2012**, *111*, 1127–1135.
619. Panagiotakopulu, E. Dipterous remains and archaeological interpretation. *J. Arch. Sci.* **2004**, *31*, 1675–1684.
620. Amendt, J.; Campobasso, C.P.; Gaudry, E.; Reiter, C.; Leblanc, H.N.; Hall, M.J. Best practice in forensic entomology-standards and guidelines. *Int. J. Leg. Med.* **2007**, *121*, 90–104.
621. Kenward, H. *Northern Regional Review of Environmental Archaeology: Invertebrates in Archaeology in the North of England: Environmental Studies Report*; English Heritage Research Department, Fort Cumberland: Swindon, UK, 2009.
622. Buckland, P.I.; Buckland, P.C.; Olsson, F. Paleoentomology: Insects and other arthropods in environmental archaeology. In *Encyclopedia of Global Archaeology*; Smith, C., Ed.; Springer: New York, NY, USA, 2014.
623. King, G.A.; Gilbert, M.T.; Willerslev, E.; Collins, M.J.; Kenward, H. Recovery of DNA from archaeological insect remains: First results, problems and potential. *J. Archaeol. Sci.* **2009**, *36*, 1179–1183.
624. Turchetto, M.; Vanin, S. Climate change and Forensic entomology. In *Current Concepts in Forensic Entomology*; Amendt, J., Campobasso, C.P., Goff, M.L., Grassberger, M., Eds.; Springer: Dordrecht, The Netherlands, 2010; pp. 327–352.
625. Prado e Castro, C.; García, M.D. First record of *Chrysomya megacephala* (Fabricius, 1794) (Diptera, Calliphoridae) from Portugal. *Graellsia* **2009**, *65*, 75–77.

626. Ebejer, M.J. The ocurrence of *Chrysomya megacephala* (Fabricius) (Diptera: Brachycera) in Malta and records of other Calliphoridae from Maltese Island. *Entomol. Mon. Mag.* **2007**, *143*, 165–170.

627. Martínez-Sánchez, A.; Ivorra, T.; Roberts, L.C.; Giner, S.; Beringola, L.M.; Cano, P.M.; Rojo, S. First record of *Chrysomya megacephala* (Diptera: Calliphoridae) on human corpses from Europe. In Proceedings of the 19th Meeting European Association of Forensic Entomology, Kolymbari, Greece, 17–20 May 2023.

628. Hochkirch, A.; Casino, A.; Penev, L.; Allen, D.; Tilley, L.; Georgiev, T.; Gospodinov, K.; Barov, B. *European Red List of Insect Taxonomists*; Publication Office of the European Union: Luxembourg, 2022.

629. Tuccia, F.; Giordani, G.; Vanin, S. A general review of the most common COI primers for Calliphoridae identification in forensic entomology. *Forensic Sci. Int. Genet.* **2016**, *24*, e9–e11.

630. Tuccia, F.; Giordani, G.; Vanin, S. A combined protocol for identification of maggots of forensic interest. *Sci. Justice* **2016**, *56*, 264–268.

631. Hebert, P.D.; Ratnasingham, S.; De Waard, J.R. Barcoding animal life: Cytochrome C Oxidase subunit 1 divergences among closely related species. *Proc. Roy. Soc. Lond. Ser. B Biol. Sci.* **2003**, *270*, S96–S99.

632. Gilarriortua, M.; Salona Bordas, M.I.; Kohnemann, S.; Pfeiffer, H.; De Pancorbo, M.M. Molecular differentiation of central European blowfly species (Diptera, Calliphoridae) using mitochondrial and nuclear genetic markers. *Forensic Sci. Int.* **2014**, *242*, 274–282.

633. Folmer, O.; Black, M.; Hoeh, W.; Lutz, R.; Vrijenhoek, R. DNA primers for amplification of mitochondrial Cytochrome C Oxidase subunit I from diverse metazoan invertebrates. *Mol. Mar. Biol. Biotech.* **1994**, *3*, 294–299.

634. Yeo, D.; Srivathsan, A.; Meier, R. Longer is not always better: Optimizing barcode length for large-scale species discovery and identification. *Syst. Biol.* **2020**, *69*, 999–1015.
635. Grzywacz, A.; Wyborska, D.; Piwczyński, M. DNA barcoding allows identification of European Fanniidae (Diptera) of forensic interest. *For. Sci. Int.* **2017**, *278*, 106–114.
636. Jordaens, K.; Sonet, G.; Richet, R.; Dupont, E.; Braet, Y.; Desmyter, S. Identification of forensically important *Sarcophaga* species (Diptera: Sarcophagidae) using the mitochondrial COI gene. *Int. J. Leg. Med.* **2013**, *127*, 491–504.
637. Gilarriortua, M.; Salona-Bordas, M.I.; Caine, L.M.; Pinheiro, F.; De Pancorbo, M.M. Mitochondrial and nuclear DNA approaches for reliable identification of Lucilia (Diptera, Calliphoridae) species of forensic interest from Southern Europe. *For. Sci. Int.* **2015**, *257*, 393–397.
638. Boheme, P.; Amendt, J.; Zehner, R. The use of COI barcodes for molecular identification of forensically important fly species in Germany. *Parasitol. Res.* **2011**, *110*, 2325–2332.
639. Gilarriortua, M.; Salona Bordas, M.I.; Caine, L.M.; Pinheiro, F.; De Pancorbo, M.M. Cytochrome b as a useful tool for the identification of blowflies of forensic interest (Diptera, Calliphoridae). *Forensic Sci. Int.*, **2013**, *228*, 132–136.
640. Giraldo, H.P.A.; Uribe, S.S.I.; Lopez, R.A. Analysis of mitochondrial DNA sequences (Cytb and ND1) in *Lucilia eximia* (Diptera: Calliphoridae). *Rev. Colomb. Entomol.* **2011**, *37*, 273–278.

641. Zehner, R.; Amendt, J.; Schütt, S.; Sauer, J.; Krettek, R.; Povolný, D. Genetic identification of forensically important flesh flies (Diptera: Sarcophagidae). *Int. J. Leg. Med.*, **2004**, *118*, 245–247.

642. Bortolini, S.; Giordani, G.; Tuccia, F.; Maistrello, L.; Vanin, S. Do longer sequences improve the accuracy of identification of forensically important Calliphoridae species? *Peer J*, **2018**, *6*, e5962.

643. McDonagh, L.M.; Stevens, J.R. The molecular systematics of blowflies and screwworm flies (Diptera: Calliphoridae) using 28S rRNA, COX1 and EF-1α: Insights into the evolution of dipteran parasitism. *Parasitology* **2011**, *138*, 1760–1777.

644. Yusseff-Vanegas, S.Z.; Agnarsson, I. DNA-barcoding of forensically important blow flies (Diptera: Calliphoridae) in the Caribbean Region. *Peer J*, **2017**, *5*, e3516.

645. Guo, Y.; Zha, L.; Yan, W.; Li, P.; Cai, J.; Wu, L. Identification of forensically important sarcophagid flies (Diptera: Sarcophagidae) in China based on COI and Period gene. *Int. J. Leg. Med.* **2014**, *128*, 221–228.

646. Schoofs, K.R.; Krzeminska Ahmadzai, U.; Goodwin, W. Analysis of the complete mitochondrial genomes of two forensically important blowfly species: *Lucilia caesar* and *Lucilia illustris*. *Mitochondrial DNA B Resour.* **2018**, *3*, 1114–1116.

647. Tautz, D.; Arctander, P.; Minelli, A.; Thomas, R.H.; Volger, A.P. A plea for DNA taxonomy. *Trends Ecol. Evol.* **2003**, *18*, 70–74.

648. Ratnasingham, S.; Hebert, P.D.N. BOLD: The Barcode of Life Data System (**www.barcodinglife.org**). *Mol. Ecol. Notes* **2007**, *7*, 355–364.

649. Glocke, I.; Meyer, M. Extending the spectrum of DNA sequences retrieved from ancient bones and teeth. *Genome Res.* **2017**, *27*, 1230–1237.

650. Reiss, R.A. Ancient DNA from ice age insects: Proceed with caution. *Quat. Sci. Rev.* 2006, *25*, 1877–1893.
651. Austin, J.J.; Smith, A.B.; Thomas, R.H. Paleontology in a molecular world: The search for authentic ancient DNA. *Tree* 1997, *12*, 303–306.
652. Fulton, T.L.; Stiller, M. 2012. PCR amplification, cloning, and sequencing of ancient DNA. *Mol. Biol.* 2012, *840*, 111–119.
653. Hofreiter, H.; Serre, D.; Poinar, H.N.; Kuch, M.; Pääbo, S. Ancient DNA. *Nat. Rev. Genet.* 2001, *2*, 353–359.
654. Hofreiter, M.; Jaenicke, V.; Serre, D.; Haeseler, A.V.; Pääbo, S. DNA sequences from multiple amplifications reveal artifacts induced by cytosine deamination in ancient DNA. *Nucleic Acids Res.* 2001, *29*, 4793–4799.
655. Smith, C.I.; Chamberlain, A.T.; Riley, M.S.; Stringer, C.; Collins, M.J. The thermal history of human fossils and the likelihood of successful DNA amplification. *J. Hum. Evol.* 2003, *45*, 203–217.
656. Handt, O.; Höss, M.; Krings, M.; Pääbo, S. Ancient DNA: Methodological challenges. *Experientia* 1994, *50*, 524–529.
657. Pedersen, M.W.; Overballe-Petersen, S.; Ermini, L.; Sarkissian, C.D.; Haile, J.; Hellstrom, M.; Spens, J.; Thomsen, P.F.; Bohmann, K.; Cappellini, E.; et al. Ancient and modern environmental DNA. Philos. *Trans. R. Soc. Lond. B Biol. Sci* 2015, *370*, 20130383.
658. Yang, D.Y.; Watt, K. Contamination controls when preparing archaeological remains for ancient DNA analysis. *J. Archaeol. Sci.* 2005, *32*, 331–336.
659. Wilson, I.G. Inhibition and facilitation of nucleic acid amplification. *Appl. Environ. Microbiol.* 1997, *63*, 3741–3751.

660. Benbow, M.E.; Tomberlin, J.K.; Tarone, A.M. *Carrion Ecology, Evolution, and Their Applications*; CRC Press: Boca Raton, FL, USA, 2015.

661. Rahi, G.S.; Adams, J.L.; Yuan, J.; Devone, D.J.; Lodhi, K.M. Whole human blood DNA degradation associated with artificial ultraviolet and solar radiations as a function of exposure time. *Forensic Sci. Int.* 2021, *319*, 110674.

662. Mcgregor, D.P.; Forster, S.; Steven, J.; Adair, J.; Leary, S.E.C.; Leslie, D.L.; Harris, W.J.; Titball, R.W. Simultaneous detection of microorganisms in soil suspension based on PCR amplification of bacterial 16S rRNA fragments. *BioTechniques* 1996, *21*, 463–471.

663. Kemp, B.M.; Monroe, C.; Smith, D.G. Repeat silica extraction: A simple technique for the removal of PCR inhibitors from DNA extracts. *J. Arch. Sci.* 2006, 33, 1680–1689.

664. Golebiowski, M. Comparison of free fatty acids composition of cuticular lipids of *Calliphora vicina* larvae and pupae. *Lipids* 2012, *47*, 1001–1009.

665. Ye, G.; Li, K.; Zhu, J.; Zhu, G.; Hu, C. Cuticular hydrocarbon composition in pupal exuviae for taxonomic differentiation of six necrophagous flies. *J. Med. Entomol.* 2007, *44*, 450–456.

666. Golebiowski, M.; Cerkowniak, M.; Bogus, M.I.; Wloka, E.; Przybysz, E.; Stepnowski, P. Developmental changes in the sterol composition and the glycerol content of cuticular and internal lipids of three species of flies. *Chem. Biodivers.* 2013, *10*, 1521–1530.

667. Golebiowski, M.; Urbanek, A.; Oleszczak, A.; Dawgul, M.; Kamysz, W.; Boguś, M.I.; Stepnowski, P. The antifungal activity of fatty acids of all stages of *Sarcophaga carnaria* L. (Diptera: Sarcophagidae). *Microbiol. Res.* 2014, *169*, 279–286.

668. Frederickx, C.; Dekeirsschieter, J.; Brostaux, Y.; Wathelet, J.P.; Verheggen, F.J.; Haubruge, E. Volatile organic compounds released by blowfly larvae and pupae: New perspectives in forensic entomology. *Forensic Sci. Int.* 2012, *219*, 215–220.
669. Kranz, W.; Carroll, C.; Dixon, D.A.; Goodpaster, J.V.; Picard, C.J. Factors affecting species identifications of blowfly pupae based upon chemical profiles and multivariate statistics. *Insects*, 2017, *8*, 43.
670. Giordani, G.; Whitmore, D.; Vanin, S. A New, non-invasive methodology for the molecular identification of adult Sarcophagidae from collections. *Insects*, 2023, *14*, 635.
671. Giordani, G.; Whitmore, D.; Vanin, S. A New, non-invasive methodology for the molecular identification of adult Sarcophagidae from collections. *Insects*, 2023, *14*, 635.
672. Chanda P, Joshi SR. Understanding the small world: the microbes. In: Verma P, editor. Industrial microbiology and biotechnology. Berlin: *Springer*; 2022, p.1–61.
673. Liu YX, Qin Y, Chen T, Lu M, Qian X, Guo X, *et al*. A practical guide to amplicon and metagenomic analysis of microbiome data. *Protein Cell*, 2021; 12: 315–30.
674. Hood L. Tackling the microbiome. *Science*, 2012; 336:1209.
675. Turnbaugh PJ, Ley RE, Hamady M, Fraser-Liggett CM, KnightR, Gordon JI. The human microbiome project: exploring the microbial part of ourselves in a changing world. *Nature*, 2007; 449:804–10.
676. Peterson J, Garges S, Giovanni M, McInnes P, Wang L, SchlossJA, *et al*. The NIH Human Microbiome Project. *Genome Res*, 2009; 19:2317–23.

677. Gilbert JA, Jansson JK, Knight R. The Earth Microbiome Project: successes and aspirations. *BMC Biol*, 2014; 12:69.
678. Fierer N, Lauber CL, Zhou N, McDonald D, Costello EK, KnightR. Forensic identification using skin bacterial communities. *Proc Nat Acad Sci U S A,* 2010; 107:6477–81.
679. Gilbert JA, Blaser MJ, Caporaso JG, Jansson JK, Lynch SV, Knight R. Current understanding of the human microbiome. *Nat Med*, 2018; 24:392–400.
680. Morgan XC, Segata N, Huttenhower C. Biodiversity and functional genomics in the human microbiome. *Trends Genet*, 2013; 29:51–8.
681. Martiny JBH, Bohannan BJM, Brown JH, Colwell RK, FuhrmanJA, Green JL, *et al*. Microbial biogeography: putting microorganisms on the map. *Nat Rev Microbiol* 2006; 4:102–12.
682. Gouello A, Dunyach-Remy C, Siatka C, Lavigne JP, *et al*.Analysis of microbial communities: an emerging tool in forensic sciences. *Diagnostics*, 2021; 12:1.
683. Metcalf JL, Xu ZZ, Bouslimani A, Dorrestein P, Carter DO, Knight R. Microbiome tools for forensic science. *Trends Biotechnol*, 2017; 35:814–23.
684. Budowle B, Schutzer SE, Einseln A, Kelley LC, Walsh AC, SmithJAL, *et al*. Public health. building microbial forensics as a response to bioterrorism. *Science*, 2003; 301:1852–3.
685. Schmedes SE, Sajantila A, Budowle B. Expansion of microbial forensics. *J Clin Microbiol*, 2016;54:1964–74.
686. Cummings CA, Chung CAB, Fang R, Barker M, Brzoska P, Williamson PC, *et al*. Accurate, rapid and high-throughput detection of strain-specific

polymorphisms in *Bacillus anthracis* and Yersinia pestis by next-generation sequencing. Investig Genet, 2010;1:5.

687. Kuleshov V, Jiang C, Zhou W, Jahanbani F, Batzoglou S, Snyder M. Synthetic long read sequencing reveals the composition and intraspecies diversity of the human microbiome. *Nat Biotechnol*, 2016; 34: 64–9.
688. Børsting C, Morling N. Next generation sequencing and its applications in forensic genetics. *Forensic Sci Int Genet*, 2015;18:78–89.
689. Budowle B, Schmedes SE, Wendt FR. Increasing the reach of forensic genetics with massively parallel sequencing. *Forensic Sci Med Pathol*, 2017; 13: 342–9.
690. Oliveira M, Amorim A. Microbial forensics: new breakthroughs and future prospects. *Appl Microbiol Biotechnol*, 2018;102:10377–91.
691. Metcalf JL, Xu ZZ, Weiss S, Lax S, Van Treuren W, Hyde ER,et al. Microbial community assembly and metabolic function during mammalian corpse decomposition. *Science*, 2016; 351:158–62.
692. Ravi RK, Walton K, Khosroheidari M. MiSeq: a next-generation sequencing platform for genomic analysis. *Methods Mol Biol*, 2018;1706: 223–32.
693. Benıtez-Paez A, Sanz Y. Multi-locus and long amplicon sequencing approach to study microbial diversity at species level using theMinIONTM portable nanopore sequencer. *Gigascience*, 2017; 6: 1–12.
694. Wagner J, Coupland P, Browne HP, Lawley TD, Francis SC, Parkhill J. Evaluation of PacBio sequencing for full-lengthbacterial 16S rRNA gene classification. *BMC Microbiol*, 2016;16: 274.

695. Tozzo P, D'Angiolella G, Brun P, Castagliuolo I, Gino S, Caenazzo L. Skin microbiome analysis for forensic human identification: What do we know so far?; *Microorganisms*, 2020; 8: 873.

696. Hillmann B, Al-Ghalith GA, Shields-Cutler RR, Zhu Q, GohlDM, Beckman KB, *et al*. Evaluating the information content of shallow shotgun metagenomics. *mSystems*, 2018; 3: e00069-18.

697. Johnson JS, Spakowicz DJ, Hong BY, Petersen LM, DemkowiczP, Chen L, *et al*. Evaluation of 16S rRNA gene sequencing for species and strain-level microbiome analysis. *Nat* Commun, 2019; 10: 5029.

698. Prodan A, Tremaroli V, Brolin H, Zwinderman AH, NieuwdorpM, Levin E. Comparing bioinformatic pipelines for microbial 16S rRNA amplicon sequencing. *PLoS One*, 2020; 15: e0227434.

699. Schloss PD, Westcott SL, Ryabin T, Hall JR, Hartmann M, Hollister EB, et al. Introducing mothur: open-source, platform independent, community-supported software for describing and comparing microbial communities. *Appl Environ Microbiol*, 2009; 75: 7537–41.

700. Caporaso JG, Kuczynski J, Stombaugh J, Bittinger K, Bushman FD, Costello EK, *et al*. QIIME allows analysis of high-throughput community sequencing data. *Nat Methods*, 2010;7:335–6.

701. Bolyen E, Rideout JR, Dillon MR, Bokulich NA, Abnet CC, Al-Ghalith GA, et al. Reproducible, interactive, scalable and extensible microbiome data science using QIIME 2. *Nat Biotechnol*, 2019; 37: 852–7.

702. Edgar RC. Search and clustering orders of magnitude faster than BLAST. *Bioinformatics*, 2010;26:2460–1.

703. Rognes T, Flouri T, Nichols B, Quince C, Mahe´ F. VSEARCH: a versatile open source tool for metagenomics. *Peer J*, 2016; 4: e2584.

704. Quast C, Pruesse E, Yilmaz P, Gerken J, Schweer T, Yarza P, *et al.* The SILVA ribosomal RNA gene database project: improved data processing and web-based tools. Nucleic Acids Res, 2013;41: D590–6.

705. DeSantis TZ, Hugenholtz P, Larsen N, Rojas M, Brodie EL, Keller K, *et al.* Greengenes, a chimera-checked 16S rRNA gene database and workbench compatible with ARB. *Appl Environ Microbiol*, 2006; 72: 5069–72.

706. Abarenkov K, Nilsson RH, Larsson KH, Alexander IJ, EberhardtU, Erland S, et al. The UNITE database for molecular identification of fungi — recent updates and future perspectives. *NewPhytol*, 2010; 186: 281–5.

707. Quince C, Walker AW, Simpson JT, Loman NJ, Segata N.Shotgun metagenomics, from sampling to analysis. *Nat Biotechnol*, 2017; 35:833–44.

708. McIver LJ, Abu-Ali G, Franzosa EA, Schwager R, Morgan XC,Waldron L, *et al.* bioBakery: a meta'omic analysis environment. *Bioinformatics*, 2018; 34: 1235–7.

709. Bolger AM, Lohse M, Usadel B. Trimmomatic: a flexible trimmerfor Illumina sequence data. *Bioinformatics*, 2014; 30: 2114–20.

710. Bharti R, Grimm DG. Current challenges and best-practice protocols for microbiome analysis. *Brief Bioinform*, 2021; 22: 178–93.

711. Truong DT, Franzosa EA, Tickle TL, Scholz M, Weingart G,Pasolli E, et al. MetaPhlAn2 for enhanced metagenomic taxonomic profiling. *Nat Methods*, 2015;12: 902–3.

712. Wood DE, Lu J, Langmead B. Improved metagenomic analysiswith Kraken 2. *Genome Biol*, 2019; 20: 257.

713. Franzosa EA, McIver LJ, Rahnavard G, Thompson LR,Schirmer M, Weingart G, et al. Species-level functional profiling of metagenomes and metatranscriptomes. *Nat Methods*, 2018; 15: 962–8.

714. Huson DH, Auch AF, Qi J, Schuster SC. MEGAN analysis ofmetagenomic data. *Genome Res*, 2007; 17: 377–86.

715. Li D, Liu CM, Luo R, Sadakane K, Lam TW. MEGAHIT: anultra-fast single-node solution for large and complex metagenomics assembly via succinct de Bruijn graph. *Bioinformatics*, 2015; 31: 1674–6.

716. Nurk S, Meleshko D, Korobeynikov A, Pevzner PA. metaSPAdes: a new versatile metagenomic assembler. *Genome Res*, 2017; 27: 824–34.

717. Zhu W, Lomsadze A, Borodovsky M. Ab initio gene identification in metagenomic sequences. *Nucleic Acids Res*, 2010; 38: e132

718. Seemann T. Prokka: rapid prokaryotic genome annotation. *Bioinformatics*, 2014; 30: 2068–9.

719. Clarke TH, Gomez A, Singh H, Nelson KE, Brinkac LM. Integrating the microbiome as a resource in the forensics toolkit. *Forensic Sci Int Genet*, 2017; 30: 141–7.

720. Alan G, Sarah JP. Microbes as forensic indicators. *Trop Biomed*, 2012; 29: 311–30.

721. Alonso A, Barrio PA, Mu¨ ller P, Ko¨ cher S, Berger B, Martin P, *et al.* Current state-of-art of STR sequencing in forensic genetics. *Electrophoresis*, 2018; 39: 2655–68.

722. Stanley UN, Khadija AM, Bukola AT, Precious IO, Davidson EA. Forensic DNA profiling: autosomal short tandem repeat as a prominent marker in crime investigation. *Malays J Med Sci*, 2020; 27: 22–35.

723. Sender R, Fuchs S, Milo R. Revised estimates for the number of human and bacteria cells in the body. *PLoS Biol*, 2016;14: e1002533.
724. Human Microbiome Project Consortium. Structure, function and diversity of the healthy human microbiome. *Nature*,2012;486:207–14.
725. Human Microbiome Project Consortium. A framework for human microbiome research. *Nature*, 2012; 486: 215–21.
726. Franzosa EA, Huang K, Meadow JF, Gevers D, Lemon KP, Bohannan BJM, *et al*. Identifying personal microbiomes using metagenomic codes. *Proc Nat Acad Sci USA*, 2015; 112: E2930–8.
727. Neckovic A, van Oorschot RAH, Szkuta B, Durdle A. Investigation into the presence and transfer of microbiomes within a forensic laboratory setting. *Forensic Sci Int Genet*, 2021; 52: 102492.
728. Dowd JB, Renson A. ''Under the skin'' and into the gut: social epidemiology of the microbiome. *Curr Epidemiol Rep*, 2018; 5: 432–41.
729. Neckovic A, van Oorschot RAH, Szkuta B, Durdle A. Investigation of direct and indirect transfer of microbiomes between individuals. *Forensic Sci Int Genet*, 2020; 45: 102212.
730. Williams DW, Gibson G. Classification of individuals and the potential to detect sexual contact using the microbiome of the pubic region. *Forensic Sci Int Genet*, 2019; 41: 177–87.
731. Lax S, Hampton-Marcell JT, Gibbons SM, Colares GB, Smith D,Eisen JA, et al. Forensic analysis of the microbiome of phones and shoes. *Microbiome*, 2015; 3: 21.
732. Meadow JF, Altrichter AE, Bateman AC, Stenson J, Brown GZ, Green JL, *et al*. Humans differ in their personal microbial cloud. *Peer J*, 2015; 3: e1258.

733. Schmedes SE, Woerner AE, Novroski NM, Wendt FR, King JL, Stephens KM, *et al.* Targeted sequencing of clade-specific markers from skin microbiomes for forensic human identification. *Forensic Sci Int Genet*, 2018; 32:50–61.
734. Woerner AE, Novroski NM, Wendt FR, Ambers A, Wiley R, Schmedes SE, et al. Forensic human identification with targeted microbiome markers using nearest neighbor classification. *Forensic Sci Int Genet*, 2019; 38: 130–9.
735. Sherier AJ, Woerner AE, Budowle B. Determining informative microbial single nucleotide polymorphisms for human identification. *Appl Environ Microbiol*, 2022; 88: e0005222.
736. Toyomane K, Yokota R, Watanabe K, Akutsu T, Asahi A, Kubota S. Optimization of microbial DNA extraction from human skin samples for CRISPR typing. *Forensic Sci Int Rep*,2022; 5: 100259.
737. Toyomane K, Yokota R, Watanabe K, Akutsu T, Asahi A, Kubota S. Evaluation of CRISPR diversity in the human skin microbiome for personal identification. *mSystems* 2021; 6: e01255-20.
738. Wilkins D, Leung MHY, Lee PKH. Microbiota fingerprints lose individually identifying features over time. *Microbiome*, 2017; 5: 1.
739. Wilkins D, Tong X, Leung MHY, Mason CE, Lee PKH. Diurnal variation in the human skin microbiome affects accuracy of forensic microbiome matching. *Microbiome*, 2021; 9:129.
740. Ruffell A. Forensic pedology, forensic geology, forensic geoscience, geoforensics and soil forensics. *Forensic Sci Int*, 2010; 202: 9–12.

741. Jesmok EM, Hopkins JM, Foran DR. Next-generation sequencing of the bacterial 16S rRNA gene for forensic soil comparison: a feasibility study. *J Forensic Sci*, 2016; 61: 607–17.

742. Trivedi M, Branton A, Trivedi D, Nayak G, Gangwar M, Jana S.Bacterial identification using 16S rDNA gene sequencing and antibiogram analysis on biofield treated Pseudomonas fluorescens. *Clin Med Biochemistry* Open Access, 2015;1: 1000101.

743. Macdonald CA, Ang R, Cordiner SJ, Horswell J. Discrimination of soils at regional and local levels using bacterial and fungal TRFLPprofiling. *J Forensic Sci*, 2011; 56: 61–9.

744. Lerner A, Shor Y, Vinokurov A, Okon Y, Jurkevitch E. Candenaturing gradient gel electrophoresis (DGGE) analysis of amplified 16S rDNA of soil bacterial populations be used in forensic investigations? *Soil Biol Biochem*, 2006; 38:1188–92.

745. Habtom H, Pasternak Z, Matan O, Azulay C, Gafny R, Jurkevitch E. Applying microbial biogeography in soil forensics.*Forensic Sci Int Genet*, 2019; 38:195–203.

746. Habtom H, Demane`che S, Dawson L, Azulay C, Matan O, RobeP, et al. Soil characterisation by bacterial community analysis for forensic applications: a quantitative comparison of environmental technologies. *Forensic Sci Int Genet* 2017; 26: 21–9.

747. Demane`che S, Schauser L, Dawson L, Franqueville L, Simonet P. Microbial soil community analyses for forensic science: application to a blind test. *Forensic Sci Int* 2017; 270: 153–8.

748. Yang T, Shi Y, Zhu J, Zhao C, Wang J, Liu Z, *et al.* The spatial variation of soil bacterial community assembly processes affects the accuracy of source tracking in ten major Chinese cities. *Sci China Life Sci*, 2021;64:1546–59.

749. Lilje L, Lillsaar T, Ra¨ tsep R, Simm J, Aaspollu A. Soil sample metagenome NGS data management for forensic investigation. *Forensic Sci Int Genet Supp* 2013; 4: e35–6.

750. Giampaoli S, Berti A, Maggio RMD, Pilli E, Valentini A, Valeriani F, *et al.* The environmental biological signature: NGSprofiling for forensic comparison of soils. *Forensic Sci Int*, 2014; 240: 41–7.

751. Danko D, Bezdan D, Afshin EE, Ahsanuddin S, Bhattacharya C, Butler DJ, *et al.* A global metagenomic map of urban microbiome and antimicrobial resistance. *Cell*, 2021; 184:3376–93.

752. Alsulimani, A.; Akhter, N.; Jameela, F.; Ashgar, R.I.; Jawed, A.; Hassani, M.A.; Dar, S.A. The Impact of Artificial Intelligence on Microbial Diagnosis. *Microorganisms*, 2024, 12, 1051. https://doi.org/10.3390/microorganisms12061051

753. Wankhade TD, Ingale SW, Mohite PM, Bankar NJ. Artificial Intelligence in Forensic Medicine and Toxicology: The Future of Forensic Medicine. *Cureus*. 2022 Aug 25;14(8): e28376. doi: 10.7759/cureus.28376. PMID: 36168339; PMCID: PMC9506671.

754. Volonnino G, De Paola L, Spadazzi F, Serri F, Ottaviani M, Zamponi MV, Arcangeli M, La Russa R. Artificial intelligence and future perspectives in Forensic Medicine: a systematic review. *Clin Ter*. 2024 May-Jun;175(3):193-202. doi: 10.7417/CT.2024.5062. PMID: 38767078.

755. Zhang X, Zhang D, Zhang X, Zhang X. Artificial intelligence applications in the diagnosis and treatment of bacterial infections. *Front Microbiol.*

2024 Aug 6; 15:1449844. doi: 10.3389/fmicb.2024.1449844. PMID: 39165576; PMCID: PMC11334354.

About Authors

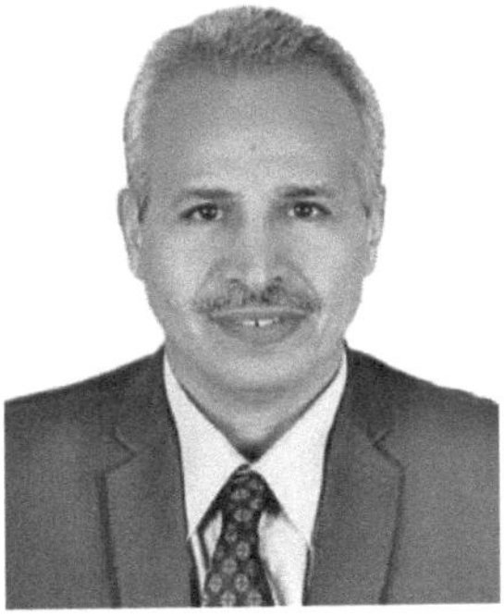

Prof. Dr. Mohamed Abdel-Raheem Ali Abdel-Raheem
Professor of Biological Control
Pests & Plant Protection Department
Agricultural and Biological Research Institute
National Research Centre.

Prof. Dr. Mohamed Abdel-Raheem Ali Abdel-Raheem, Prof. of Entomology (Biological Control), Pests & Plant Protection Department, Agricultural and Biological Research Institute, National Research Centre, Cairo, Egypt. Published publications (302) papers (82), Books and Book chapters (220), (Scopus) h-index (11), Citations (299), (Google Scholar) h-index (19) , Citations (1070), (Web of Science) Publications (9), h-index (5), Citations (51), Research Gate, h-index

(14), Citations (646), Reviewers in International Journals (139), Reviewed articles in Biological Control (812), Editor in Chief in Journal (7), Editorial board in Journals (35), Associated Editor in Chief in Journal (5), Advisory board (1), conference Attended (27), workshop Attended (293), Symposium Attended (176), Forum Attended (4), Prize (4), Attended Others (30), Projects As PI and member (19), Training courses For Agric. Engineering (61), Training courses For Students of University (8), attending Trainees courses (19), TV, Radio & Newspaper (26), Supervisor on Ph.D. thesis (1), Committee Ph.D. thesis (2), and member in scientific Foundation (14), Giving International lectures (3).

National Research Centre. 33rd ElBohouth St., Dokki, Cairo, Egypt.

Email Address: abdelraheem_nrc@hotmail.com, ma.abdel-raheem@nrc.sci.eg, abdelraheem_nrc@yahoo.com, profmohamedabdelraheem@gmail.com, abdelraheem196942@gmail.com, Mohamedabdelraheem42@gmail.com, Mabdelraheem69@gmail.com, mohamed196942@yahoo.com, mabdel-raheem@hotmil.com,

Mobile Phone: (+2) 01155527583 – (+2) 01009580797

Scopus Author ID : 55220661700

https://www.scopus.com/authid/detail.uri?authorId=55220661700

http://scholar.google.com/citations?hl=en&user=gBtssEgAAAAJ

https://orcid.org/my-orcid?orcid=0000-0001-9240-064X

https://www.webofscience.com/wos/author/searchAbdel-Raheem, Mohamed Abdel-Raheem Ali - Web of Science Core Collection

https://www.researchgate.net/profile/Mohamed_Abdel-Raheem4/publications?sorting=recentlyAdded

http://livedna.org/20.16018

http://www.resarcherid.com/rid/R-6264-2017

https://www.webofscience.com/wos/author/record/R-6264-2017
https://www.facebook.com/share/p/1Piu6xyFmN/

- TV, Radio & Newspaper

1. https://www.youtube.com/attribution_link?a=NsH2xGv9mY8&u=%2Fwatch%3Fv%3Dsb46rBG8-Mc%26feature%3Dshare
2. https://youtu.be/Ub8djW0tggo
3. https://m.facebook.com/story.php?story_fbid=492907069288338&id=100076011247165
4. https://youtu.be/dOujUAZmTdw
5. https://m.facebook.com/story.php?story_fbid=492907069288338&id=100076011247165
6. https://fb.watch/gPGrDuzZFX/
7. https://www.youtube.com/watch?si=4UfyQaeHVLPiVR5J&v=nXV4NT-no7o&feature=youtu.be
8. https://www.youtube.com/watch?v=sRH44W6TbcQ
9. https://youtu.be/uq9Qj3AEBHk?si=ymaX06huG2AXJESu
10. https://www.facebook.com/share/v/Qg5s6HW3hD8PLBzp/?mibextid=xfxF2i
11. https://el-yom.com/news/archives/1092767
12. https://el-yomnews.com/?p=1156515
13. https://el-yomnews.com/%D8%A7%D9%84%D8%AF%D9%83%D8%AA%D9%88%D8%B1-%D8%B9%D8%A8%D8%AF%D8%A7%D9%84%D8%B1%D8%AD%D9%8A%D9%85-%D9%85%D8%AD%D9%85%D8%AF-

%D8%B9%D9%84%D9%8A-
%D9%8A%D8%AA%D8%AD%D8%AF%D8%AB-%D9%84-
%D9%84%D9%84/

14. https://el-yomnews.com/?p=1179515
15. https://www.facebook.com/share/v/4MM85wKRPxsYLqTr/
16. https://el-
yomnews.com/%d8%a7%d9%84%d8%ad%d8%b4%d8%b1%d8%a7%d8%
aa-%d9%81%d9%8a-%d8%ae%d8%af%d9%85%d8%a9-
%d8%a7%d9%84%d8%b9%d8%af%d8%a7%d9%84%d8%a9-
%d9%85%d8%ad%d8%a7%d8%b6%d8%b1%d8%a9-
%d8%aa%d9%83%d8%b4%d9%81-%d8%af%d9%88/
17. https://youtube.com/watch?v=F21ziQxdeco&si=LvSUixmnSg4JM1zK
18. https://youtu.be/F21ziQxdeco?si=jyAwbU8dVwkYzRH4

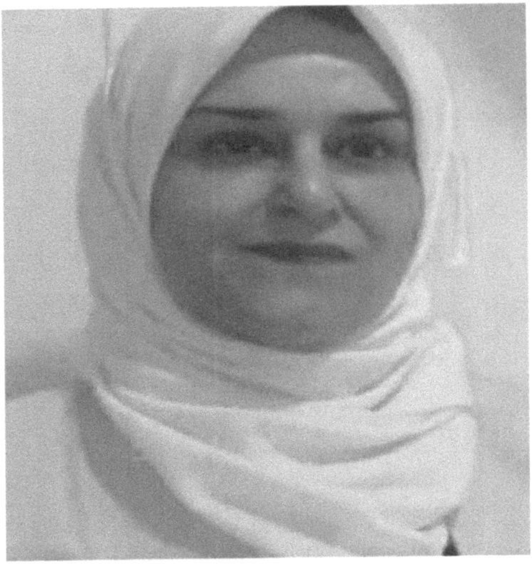

Prof. Dr. Taghreed Khudhur Muhammed

Microbiology, Bacterial Toxicology, Technical Medical Institute, Al-Mansour - Middle Technical University - Baghdad - Iraq

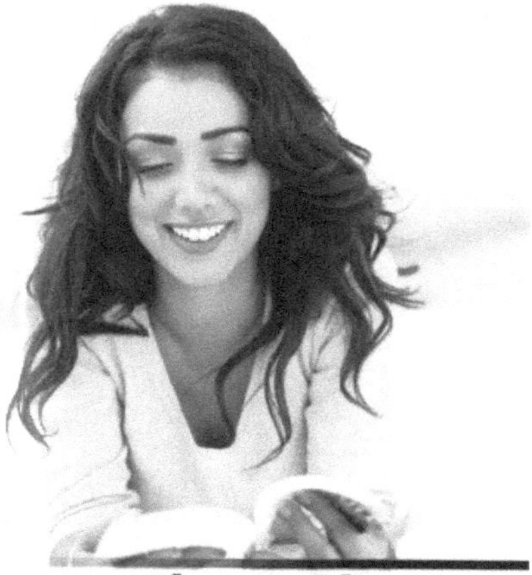

Kolibri 360 GmbH
Ferdinand-Jühlke-Straße 7
99095 Erfurt, Deutschland
produktsicherheit@kolibri360.de

Druck:
CPI Druckdienstleistungen GmbH
im Auftrag der
Kolibri 360 GmbH
Ferdinand-Jühlke-Str. 7
99095 Erfurt